Holistic Medicine
and the
Extracellular
Matrix

"Matthew Wood is among the most respected and well-known herbalists of our era and is the author of several brilliant textbooks on herbal medicine. *Holistic Medicine and the Extracellular Matrix* is his opus and masterpiece. Exceptionally well written and impeccably researched, this book debunks the popular theory that cells of the body function as independent units existing independently of one another. Instead, he meticulously reveals in easy-to-understand terms the implications of the extracellular matrix, the inner ocean in which the cells exist, and how this simple switch hugely impacts our understanding of healing. This book is a must-read for anyone interested in health, healing, and medicine."

ROSEMARY GLADSTAR, HERBALIST AND
AUTHOR OF *PLANTING THE FUTURE*

"*Holistic Medicine and the Extracellular Matrix* is a deep examination of the scientific justification of concepts discussed in traditional systems of medicine for millennia—that the human organism is a living wholeness unto itself, not a compilation of unintelligent biochemical and cellular machinery. This groundbreaking text reveals the truth of how our bodies function at a fundamental level and how we can rejuvenate our health on all levels with natural, holistic approaches to healing. It's akin to the discovery of the heliocentric model of our solar system but for the understanding and practice of holistic medicine ... truly revolutionary."

SAJAH POPHAM, AUTHOR OF *EVOLUTIONARY HERBALISM*

"Matthew Wood's book turns biomedical physiology on its head and presents a science-based holistic perspective on how and why herbs really work. His finest book yet!"

ROBERT DALE ROGERS, RH (AHG),
AUTHOR OF *ROGERS' SCHOOL OF HERBAL MEDICINE*

"In his groundbreaking book, *Holistic Medicine and the Extracellular Matrix,* Matthew Wood brings us a more balanced scientific perspective and further proves the basic tenet of holism while condemning reductionism as a model for how biological systems work. A revolutionary work poised to overthrow the conceptual foundation of modern science and its therapeutic models and drug therapies, this book directs treatment toward the individual as a whole and blows the lid off a 'one-size-fits-all' approach to modern pharmacology and compares our situation to that of Galileo and the Church. I recommend this book for all students of herbalism, holistic medicine, and the curative arts."

THEA SUMMER DEER, CLINICAL HERBALIST
AND AUTHOR OF *WISDOM OF THE PLANT DEVAS*

"Matthew Wood's brilliant new book definitively establishes the scientific basis of holistic healing. Wood shows how optimal health—homeostasis—is in the extracellular matrix, the fundamental basis of alternative medicine. Drugs circumvent the self-regulation of our bodies and are creating more diabetes, cardiovascular distress, and cancer, yet holistic therapies improve the cellular environment and our bodies' balance. I especially admire this book because Wood brings in Arthur Firstenberg's research on the intensifying electromagnetic frequencies as the cause of much modern disease. The extracellular matrix that transports our bodily fluids is very sensitive to these frequencies that may be causing the huge rise in inflammation today. This is a must-read for herbalists, acupuncturists, chiropractors, energy therapists, bodyworkers, and anyone directing their own path to healing."

BARBARA HAND CLOW, AUTHOR OF
ASTROLOGY AND THE RISING OF KUNDALINI

Holistic Medicine

and the

Extracellular Matrix

The Science of Healing
at the Cellular Level

A Sacred Planet Book

MATTHEW WOOD

Healing Arts Press
Rochester, Vermont

Healing Arts Press
One Park Street
Rochester, Vermont 05767
www.HealingArtsPress.com

Text stock is SFI certified

Healing Arts Press is a division of Inner Traditions International

Sacred Planet Books are curated by Richard Grossinger, Inner Traditions editorial board member and cofounder and former publisher of North Atlantic Books. The Sacred Planet collection, published under the umbrella of the Inner Traditions family of imprints, is comprised of works on the themes of consciousness, cosmology, alternative medicine, dreams, climate, permaculture, alchemy, shamanic studies, oracles, astrology, crystals, hyperobjects, locutions, and subtle bodies.

Note to the reader: This book is intended as an informational guide. The remedies, approaches, and techniques described herein are meant to supplement, and not to be a substitute for, professional medical care or treatment. They should not be used to treat a serious ailment without prior consultation with a qualified health care professional.

Cataloging-in-Publication Data for this title is available from the Library of Congress

ISBN 978-1-64411-294-6 (print)
ISBN 978-1-64411-295-3 (ebook)

Printed and bound in the United States by Lake Book Manufacturing, Inc. The text stock is SFI certified. The Sustainable Forestry Initiative® program promotes sustainable forest management.

10 9 8 7 6 5 4 3 2 1

Text design and layout by Priscilla H. Baker
This book was typeset in Garamond Premier Pro with Acherus Grotesque and Gill Sans used as display typeface

To send correspondence to the author of this book, mail a first-class letter to the author c/o Inner Traditions • Bear & Company, One Park Street, Rochester, VT 05767, and we will forward the communication, or contact the author directly at **www.matthewwoodinstituteofherbalism.com**.

Contents

Foreword

Stephen Harrod Buhner

*Once [reductive] science convinced us the world was dead,
it could begin its autopsy in earnest.*

JAMES HILLMAN

Anything will give up its secrets if you love it enough.

GEORGE WASHINGTON CARVER

We are in difficult times, and it's time for a change. Most people on this Earth know it. The challenges we face are demanding a significant alteration in the way we approach this planet that is our home, the lack of kindness in our culture's systemic denigration of the weak and not-rich, and how we view and treat diseases and those who are suffering from them.

In my many medical herbals, the series of ecological books culminating with *Plant Intelligence and the Imaginal Realm,* and in a number of my recent articles and blog posts, I have been arguing for the emergence of a more sophisticated and holistic approach in our relation to Earth. This includes herbal medicine (and so many other things) as well as necessitates a shift from the approach of the reductive phytorationalists who keep producing simplistic texts based on a very flawed medical model.

We are no longer in the late nineteenth or mid twentieth centuries. The world is changing and so is disease. And the pictures of the human body, this Earth, and life itself that the reductive world keeps teaching children are terribly flawed, so inaccurate in fact that it is those beliefs that are destroying the fabric of our planetary home as well as keeping alive an approach to medicine whose paradigm is not sufficient to deal with what we are now facing: the rise of antibiotic resistant diseases, viral pandemics, the emergence of ecological disruption diseases such as Lyme, as well as the massive development of chronic conditions such as long Covid.

American herbalists, of necessity, need to abandon that older medical model and actively create our own unique and sophisticated paradigm of health, plant medicines, the human body, and the role of the practitioner in healing. Regrettably, the current training of "clinical" herbalists still uses a reductive medical approach to plants, the human body, and disease, with little room for the human elements that are essential to healing, and shows as well a complete lack of awareness of the actual nature of organs, organisms, plants, and Earth (as self-organizing, nonlinear, highly intelligent, living systems displaying emergent behavior).

In fact, the more "serious and academic" herbal training has become, the worse it gets. The world doesn't need more baby doctors trying to get mom and dad to like them and let them play in the big sandbox. The medical approach to healing (except in dealing with severe physical trauma) is flawed beyond salvaging. An entirely new system needs to be created, which is what we, as herbalists, should be doing. (Those with chronic diseases such as Lyme, COPD, and long Covid already know this.)

I have long bemoaned the fact that there are so very few herbalists and texts that are pushing the envelope, that is, taking on the challenge of doing this, creating the sophisticated foundations and understandings that are necessary for a truly holistic, sophisticated healing work based around the use of plant medicines.

Few if any clinical schools, of whatever sort, train their students in establishing rapport, active listening, empathy, effective communication techniques, the psychological dynamics of disease and health, or anything else related to the human beings that come to them in their suffering. It is an egregious failure, and, frankly, contemptible. None of those programs are apparently aware of complexity theory, living organ systems, nonlinearity in living systems, ecology, or even the *extent* and importance of the human and Earth microbiomes. (We have a microbiome in our lungs denied to be in existence until a decade ago; that we have commensal bacterial populations throughout our bodies is still not widely recognized.)

In any event, before this rant gets too far out of control, I want to tell you the reason for it. Matthew Wood has written just the sort of book I have long been advocating. It's a brilliant and long overdue exploration and recognition of the extracellular matrix as an organ in its own right . . . one upon which our health depends.

The extracellular matrix (ECM) is crucial to holistic medicine because it is the foundational system from which all else springs, and it is not possible to understand physiology in a holistic fashion without understanding the ECM. Indeed, the ECM demands holism in biology and medicine because it shows us that the entire organism functions as a whole unit on the cellular level. Not just Earth-centered herbalists, but even hardened mechanists and reductionists, need to know about the matrix so that their herbalism can be founded on confident, holistic, and successful practice. Reductionism as the ruling theme in medicine can no longer be considered scientific; besides which, it has always been incapable of addressing chronic health problems or the needs of the soul and body complex.

I consider this book essential reading for all herbalists and part of the foundation for a truly sophisticated approach to the healing of disease.

Well done, Matthew!

STEPHEN HARROD BUHNER is one of the most accomplished writers on medical herbalism in the United States. He is the author of several books, including, with Inner Traditions, *Healing Lyme Disease Coinfections, Natural Treatments for Lyme Coinfections, Natural Remedies for Low Testosterone,* and *The Transformational Power of Fasting.* Stephen is also known for his numerous articles as well as for his memoir and fictional short stories and poems. He is the winner of a Nautilus Book Award and the BBC Environmental Book of the Year Award for *The Lost Language of Plants.* Stephen is an interdisciplinary, independent scholar who is a Fellow of Schumacher College and a researcher for the Foundation for Gaian Studies. His website is stephenharrodbuhner.com.

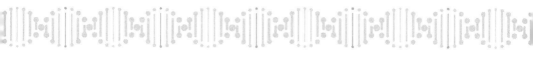

Introduction

Scientific Justification for
Holistic Medicine

*We look at the living matrix from a variety of different,
but related views. As with an elaborate sculpture, every
perspective gives a different image. . . . there are undoubtedly other perspectives we do not yet know about.*

JAMES L. OSCHMAN (2016, 169)

Before I became an herbalist, I was an artist. One of the lessons I
learned as an artist is perspective. This refers to the ability to place the
objects in the foreground in the correct relationship with those in the
background. Applying this to running our lives, we speak of "having
perspective" in life-management terms, meaning we understand which
issues are more important and which are less so. One can have a dis-
torted view of what is important in life, but in the art world lack of
perspective is a decisive matter. If one's works don't have it, it will be
obvious in some way, and the person will be seen as an amateur. This
might be acceptable, quaint, even desirable if one is a folk artist, a naïf,
or an untrained visionary, but a professional artist cannot be excused
for creating works with incorrect perspective. It is obvious and creates a
sort of distortion that is disturbing.

Just as perspective is needed in art and life, it also is required in science. Overemphasis or overfamiliarity with one fact can lead to a lack

1

of scientific perspective. This is an easy mistake to make when all the facts are not in, which is often the case in any scientific endeavor. It happens that many of the basic concepts in biology and biomedicine in place today date back to the nineteenth century, when science simply did not have enough facts to establish perspective.

Not infrequently, it is supposed that all the facts are in and that the perspective derived from them is correct. This can lead to a mistake becoming so entrenched that it becomes a "truth" when in fact it is completely wrong. This is a problem with the modern understanding of the extracellular matrix (ECM) and the cell. The cell theory of Rudolf Virchow (1821–1902) has been in vogue for so long, since the mid-nineteenth century, that it is impossible for most people to think of the cell as anything but the ultimate unit of life and an independent entity that directs its own destiny. Even now, when this theory has been proven wrong, it is still a widespread, unquestioned assumption of both the lay public and the scientific world. Here, for instance, is a typical quote from a responsible, science-based holistic site on the internet:

> Biologists who study the nature of living things typically regard the cell as the smallest functional unit of life.

I don't want to give the address of the website because it is a responsible and prominent source about holistic medicine, but I use this as an example of how entrenched this completely wrong idea is, both in conventional and alternative science and medicine.

It turns out that each cell in the body is completely controlled by the ECM around it—by its environment. Cells feed, eliminate, replicate, and migrate only when signaled to do so by the ground regulatory system (GRS), a system of communication vested in the polymers of the ECM *outside the cell.* The ultimate unit of life in higher organisms is not the cell, therefore, but the capillary/matrix/cell unit as a whole (Pischinger 2007). This means that on the cellular level, the organism functions as a whole and the cells are subordinate parts of the whole.

The discovery of the GRS by Alfred Pischinger (1903–1982) therefore proves the basic tenet of holism.

You may say, "But what about the single cell floating in the ocean? How can that not be the captain of its own ship?" Pischinger thought of this, too. He realized that the idea of a cell living by itself, independent of its environment, was impossible. Thus, he noted:

Seawater is the primary regulatory system of the single cell. (Pischinger 2007, 3)

This statement makes a great deal more sense today, when we are aware of the importance of the biome that all beings live in and the microbiome of living beings within us. The environment is the ultimate regulatory system for human and amoeba.

There is an important reason why Pischinger could understand this and others could not. He was a holistic physician and researcher at the University of Vienna Medical School. He came from a long line of physicians and researchers at that school who had resisted Virchow's cell theory from its inception. This gave him a perspective that was different from those who then—and now—remain stuck on the cell theory.

At the time of Virchow's ascendance, he was opposed by Carl von Rokitansky (1804–1878), dean of the prestigious medical school at Vienna. The latter would not agree with Virchow, and for the next four or five generations, the Vienna school carried on a quiet opposition to this theory until, at last, Pischinger proved Virchow wrong. This, to me, is a much more remarkable story of resistance to scientific blindness than, for example, that of the Church and Galileo, because it involved generations and not just an individual. Ironically, it involved a scientific blindness very similar to the resistance to geocentrism: cytocentrism.

The discovery of the GRS justifies the holistic model of medicine because it shows us that on the cellular level the organism operates as a single unit to which every cell is entirely subordinate. It equally condemns reductionism as the basis for biology and medicine, since it shows that the health of every cell is controlled by the organism as a whole. Thus, it even condemns conventional drug therapy. As Pischinger points out, directing the drug toward the receptor site on the cell membrane bypasses the GRS and therefore weakens the self-regulation of the organism. Correct treatment should be directed toward the GRS and the matrix polymers that support it. Holistic therapy has always been directed toward the whole being, not the cell, much less the individual receptor on the cell membrane.

Pischinger first published this information in English in 1975 in *Matrix and Matrix Regulation: Basis for Holistic Theory in Medicine,* yet it is still largely unknown, even by adherents of holistic medicine. This oversight is not entirely intentional: as a researcher in the field, Anna Dongari-Bagtzoglou (2008, 201), comments, "Mere visualization of the ECM has been problematic." If we train our thinking based on wrong assumptions, we cannot see correctly. We are completely unaware of our lack of perspective.

Recognition of the matrix has made some headway in certain fields. The understanding of wound healing requires knowledge of the local terrain of the ground substance that makes up the architectural structure of the matrix. The study of wound healing is, in fact, one of the easier ways to get insight into the ECM. I have, for this reason, dedicated an entire chapter to this subject—along with some herbs, the actions of which I did not fully grasp until I understood the matrix. The other area in which science has accepted and worked with the "Pischingerian" perspective is in the understanding and treatment of cancer. There are several reasons, to be pointed out in chapter 3, "The Ground Substance," why it is impossible to understand or treat some kinds of cancer without appreciating the role of the matrix in the development, containment, signaling, and expansion of those kinds of cancer. Pischinger himself already understood this before his death in 1982.

Subsequent research has shown that each organ is surrounded by its own matrix, with its own peculiar chemistry and regulatory system, and enclosed within its own serous membrane. Since the serous membrane is fairly permeable, the individual organ or tissue is not separated from the whole but contiguous with it. On the other hand, there is also an element of independence from the whole. This means that, within limitations, the organ has a life of its own. It develops through complex intercommunication within its own matrix and continues this communication throughout life (Frantz, Stewart, and Weaver 2010). This justifies the perspective of holistic medicine, which places great value not only on the whole organism but also on treatment by tissue, organ, system, or (to borrow a phrase from traditional Chinese medicine) "organ system." These are now seen to be "little wholes," operating within the greater whole of the organism, which itself operates within the greater whole of Nature. The folk medicine concept of "liver remedies" or "stomach remedies" turns out to be based on medical fact. Of course, this idea is not unfamiliar to conventional medicine, either, in which specialties are often defined by organs or systems.

If we are going to deconstruct and reconstruct the matrix, we also need to take a second look at the cell within the matrix. A new vision of the cell, compatible with Pischinger's work, was formulated by Gerald H. Pollack (2001). The two views are integrated by Elliot Overton (2018). The same principles that operate in the matrix—the presence of polymers that thicken the fluids into "glop" or "gel," with electrical charges on the polymers carrying signals—also extend to the communication system within the cell. We even need to take a look at bacteria, which communicate with each other within and through the matrix through quorum sensing, a process described in chapter 3.

An even more recent model is the cell danger response (see chapter 5). At this point, the model places the basic response in the single cell (with signaling through the matrix to adjacent cells), so this theory pushes the pendulum back toward Virchow somewhat. However, it remains impossible to now imagine the cell and its defensive responses occurring independent of the matrix. Although only a "model" at this time, I have included an account of the cell danger response, because it makes a great deal of sense. Also, it demonstrates that there may be some "push back" from the cell toward the matrix. The exact balance between the environment of the cell and the individual cell in the body can probably never be fully measured.

Pischinger understood that he had uncovered an underlying mechanism upon which to base holistic medicine. The organism acts and reacts as a whole, and no amount of reductionism—exploration down to the smallest parts—can obscure the unity observed in the action of the GRS. Pischinger also understood that his findings would be ignored. Three hundred years of reductionism plows onward, just as geocentrism plowed onward after it had been disproved. The parts continue to be set before the whole. This perspective remains in place due to habit, superficial thinking, the monetary influence of established, profit-based medicine, and professional politics. Modern research on the matrix has proceeded apace, delving into the bits and pieces of the matrix but almost entirely ignoring the holism inherent in Pischinger's discovery.

HOW DID SCIENCE LOSE THE THREAD?

The inability to perceive or understand the ECM is not a small mistake. Awareness of the ECM is as significant as the understanding of heliocentrism. It is not overly dramatic to say that biology and medicine have lost contact with a basic thread of physiological reality. How can such an oversight be explained? It is one thing to oppose holism because it is "not proved," but it is another matter to oppose holism after it has been proven to be true. One feels that science has lost the actual thread of reality.

Late in the composition of *The Extracellular Matrix,* I met holistic medical researcher Arthur Firstenberg in Santa Fe, New Mexico, and became acquainted with his unique book, *The Invisible Rainbow: The History of Electricity and Life* (2016). Up until this time, I had been a skeptic about the influence of electromagnetic frequencies (also called EMFs) on health. This is not really what I want to emphasize right now, however. Arthur purposed what I thought was a sympathetic and insightful explanation for when and where modern medicine first took a turn to delusion.

After World War II, he explained, the number of chemicals introduced into industry and science without careful study of their potential toxicity increased by the tens of thousands. Medicine faced a choice: it could either demand that these substances be studied before they were safely released into the environment, or it could knuckle under to the virtually unstoppable behemoth of power and money that was starting to rely on these substances for industry, commerce, politics, medicine, and finance. The leaders of medical science essentially had no choice but to compromise their scientific standards. The new foundation of medicine was, like the emperor's new clothes, something that could not bear close examination. This led to a dogmatic stance fiercer than what was found in the first half of the twentieth century.

"A Turn Towards Darkness"

Recently, the recognition has started to trickle into medicine that serious mistakes are being made. John Ioannidis, now a professor at Stanford University, shocked the medical community in 2005 with his examination of the weaknesses in mathematical models in biomedical research. He showed that 70 percent of papers could not possibly prove anything because they were based on flawed statistical models. His first paper, "Why Most Published Research Findings Are False," has been visited over a million times on PubMed. In another paper, Ioannidis and a coworker, Jonathan D. Schoenfeld, applied the same statistical standards to the extensive literature devoted to showing that many common foods and herbs have mutagenic properties.

> In an illustrative study, Schoenfeld and Ioannidis (2013) choose the first 50 ingredients from randomly chosen recipes from the Boston Cooking-School Cook Book, and searched the medical literature for studies linking these ingredients to various forms of cancer. For 40 of these, they found at least one study, and for

20 they found at least 10 studies. Examining the reported associations, the authors found a pattern of strong effects reported with relatively weak statistical support, with larger effect sizes reported in individual studies than in meta-analyses. In addition, they found a dramatically wide range of reported relative risks associated with an additional serving per day with each food item, well beyond what seems credible for more well-established effects. (Card and Srivastava 2014)

The authors criticized Chinese research in which the studies were looking for positive results, rather than negative ones. In China, the attempt is made to find proof for the positive effects of natural foods and herbs; in America, research often attempts to prove lack of medical value or even danger.

Some of the most commonly used tools for the person trying to make use of scientific studies are systematic reviews or meta-analyses in which major studies are lumped together and compared with each other. However, Ioannides takes on these potentially useful tools in "The Mass Production of Redundant, Misleading, and Conflicted Systematic Reviews and Meta-analysis" (Ioannides 2016). The paper found that only 3 percent of meta-analyses and reviews are both clinically useful and based on solidly constructed research.

A good review of Ioannides's work, from the layperson's viewpoint, "Lies, Damned Lies, and Medical Science," was penned by David H. Freedman (2010).

Dr. Marcia Angell, onetime editor of the *New England Journal of Medicine,* has also been heroic, coming at the issue from the standpoint of the corruptive influence of money in medicine in *The Truth about Drug Companies* (2004). Here is a comment from her:

It is simply no longer possible to believe much of the clinical research that is published, or to rely on the judgment of trusted physicians or authoritative medical guidelines. I take no pleasure in this conclusion, which I reached slowly and reluctantly over my two decades as an editor of the *New England Journal of Medicine*. (Angell 2009)

Some scientists have attempted to rectify these wrongs with papers such as "Financial Ties of Principal Investigators and Randomized Control Trial Outcomes: Cross Sectional Study" by R. Ahn and "Big Pharma Often Commits Corporate Crime, and This Must Be Stopped" by P. C. Gøtzsche.

Finally, Dr. Richard Horton, editor of the *Lancet,* gave a chilling account following a national meeting held in the United Kingdom in 2015.

"A lot of what is published is incorrect." I'm not allowed to say who made this remark because we were asked to observe Chatham House rules. We were also asked not to take photographs of slides. Those who worked for government agencies pleaded that their comments especially remain unquoted, since the forthcoming UK election meant they were living in "purdah"—a chilling state where severe restrictions on freedom of speech are placed on anyone on the government's payroll. Why the paranoid concern for secrecy and non-attribution? Because this symposium—on the reproducibility and reliability of biomedical research, held at the Wellcome Trust in London last week—touched on one of the most sensitive issues in science today: the idea that something has gone fundamentally wrong with one of our greatest human creations.

The case against science is straightforward: much of the scientific literature, perhaps half, may simply be untrue. Afflicted by studies with small sample sizes, tiny effects, invalid exploratory analyses, and flagrant conflicts of interest, together with an obsession for pursuing fashionable trends of dubious importance, science has taken a turn towards darkness. (Horton 2015)

Lack of Perspective Can Be Unintentional

Sometimes a lack of perspective seems to have nothing to do with the battle against holism, the surrender to modern industry, or the corruptive influence of drug money. Sometimes no particular reason for overlooking and ignoring important facts seems evident. I would, however, dare to say that this kind of myopia points to a lack of cultivation of critical and intuitive instincts in thinking, which would otherwise save us from bold digressions from truth and reality.

The premise that a drug must have a specific, local, molecular action on a receptor site or tissue is the cornerstone of modern drug therapy, yet it cannot be defended scientifically. Not only does this position ignore Pischinger's proof that the cell is not the regulatory center for itself, but it also flies in the face of basic facts of Nature. Roger J. Williams took this up in his book *Biochemical Individuality* (1977). He shows that every human being is unique and individual, with widely idiosyncratic and variable organ sizes and shapes, hormone levels, biochemistry, and nutritional needs. (No attempt was made to measure environmental influences, which are even more variable.) Because of this, no two individuals will *ever* react the same way to the same drug. Yet, the ideal of modern pharmacology is based on a "one-size-fits-all" model. Not only is this approach physiologically, statistically, biochemically, and functionally unfounded, but it also flies in the face of basic facts of science. As Williams comments:

> If our interpretation is correct, it will be quite impossible to find a drug that will act with complete uniformity on all human beings. In order for this to be accomplished, variation, the cornerstone of evolution, and biochemical individuality, would have to be abolished. (Williams 1977, 117)

If pharmacology and medicine oppose the theory of evolution, as well as basic physiological facts involving the control of cellular life, then we are really talking about a profound lapse in truth, reality, and effectiveness. Our situation is entirely comparable to that of Galileo and geocentrism.

THE HOLISTIC PATH

The purpose of this book is to acquaint holistic health professionals and the lay public with our new, expanding knowledge of the matrix. We not only need to know that holism is justified by scientific facts, but we also need to have textbooks written from this perspective. If we in the field do not write them, nobody else will do it for us. I am not an expert in this field, but once I understood Pischinger's research, I knew I had to explain it as a health educator and use it as a practicing herbalist. That meant I had to collect data. To do this right involved an ever-increasing corpus of knowledge that I would not, at the beginning, have thought of as related to the main premise. However, it was necessary to place the matrix within certain perspectives.

On a personal note, throughout this book I have written as a complementary and alternative medicine practitioner, breaking from accepted scientific speech intentionally. I have seeded the text freely with holistic concepts, personalities, and therapies. I have also written in a somewhat informal mode from time to time. An example of this is found in my use of the term *matrix* instead of the accepted usage of *ECM*. One of my peculiarities is the capitalization of the common names of herbs, which I picked up from herbalist Margi Flint. As she says, "Herbs are my friends so I capitalize their names, like I would my other friends."

Writing on a topic of modern scientific interest does not come to me easily. I spent the first two years of my life on the remote Seminole Indian reservation in the Everglades, where English was a second language and people had only been in a treaty relationship with the U.S. government for twenty years. This is where my language skills and mental reference points took root. The understanding embedded in that language and culture permanently shaped my thought-universe, so that for me, Western science has always been an intrinsically intrusive element.

In order for me to use the tools of Western science, I have to make clear my personal problems with this discipline. I experience Western science as a hegemonic, conceited, imbalanced system that devalues the subjective experiences of individual people as well as the cultures of whole peoples. I do not want to make this a political issue; it is simply a perspective that is important for my readers to understand about me.

Western science was founded on the idea that empathy, intuition, instinct, imagination, and other such experiences that are natural to the human species should not be trusted as means for acquiring knowledge. This has now become an assumption so deeply embedded in Western culture that it is essentially the unexamined "religion" of modern, educated people within the system. Science thinks it is somehow based on truth, whereas, in fact, it is based on an editing of experience. A balanced perspective would teach us that we have to develop all aspects of human nature and that our system of knowledge is innately incomplete unless we do.

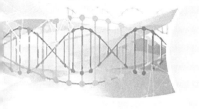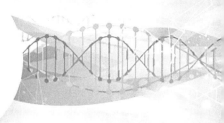

The Extracellular Matrix
The Primal Organ System

*That which formerly seemed only intended to fill up or to
form a protective covering now appears to us as the matrix
through which the most secret currents pass from the blood
to the tissues and back from these to the blood vessels, at the
same time serving as one of the most important breeding
places for young cells, which may then be raised from their
undeveloped youthful form into the most special structures
of the body.*

JACOB MOLESCHOTT
(QUOTED IN SCHÜESSLER 1898, 28)

Life began in the Great Mother Ocean of antiquity. The first living
organisms enclosed a drop of seawater and some protein chains within
a carbohydrate-lipid membrane. For this reason, the water in all living
cells has an electrolyte mix diluted but identical in proportion to the
salts found in the Great Mother Ocean of antiquity, three and a half
billion years ago.

Oceans have come and gone, leaving the different colors in the salts
that we put in our food today—pink, orange, gray, white. Having left
the Great Mother Ocean, we constantly need to take up minerals that
are no longer available to us from the original mother of life. Some of

them, such as iodine, are much more difficult to get on land than by sea, leading to diseases such as iodine-deficiency goiter.

The homeland of the first single-cell organisms was probably at the seashore, where the bright, warm sunlight beat against rocks, sands, and muds. There, early living cells received energy from the sun, gases from the air, water modified by sunshine, minerals from sea and stone, and nucleotides and carbon compounds that were created by inorganic processes but became the basis of the life process. Early on, they received help from *porphyrins,* light-sensitive substances that facilitate electron exchange, including oxidation.

Eventually, colonies of genetically identical single cells enclosed seawater within a membrane to stabilize their environment—to make it internal. Thus was born the *extracellular matrix* (ECM) surrounding the cells of multicellular organisms. But what was the precursor to this matrix?

THE PERICELLULAR MATRIX

The model for the extracellular matrix was the *pericellular matrix.* This was a polysaccharide coating around the perimeter of single-cell organisms floating in the sea that they generated to protect themselves against the buffets of the Great Mother Ocean. It turns out that this structure—composed of sugar-lipids and sugar-proteins—acts not only as a protective coating, as was first thought, but also as a medium for communication between the environment and the cell. If we draw a boundary between the cell and its environment, we would say that the cell membrane and its pericellular matrix was the "brain" of the cell, telling it what to do. However, this structure is only reacting to the outside environment, so Mother Nature is the ultimate "brain" of the cell.

These facts have a practical application. Research by Barbara A. Israel and Warren I. Schaeffer (1988) shows that when the nucleus from a cancerous cell is put in a healthy cell, the cell remains healthy. However, when the nucleus from a healthy cell is put into a cancerous cell, the cell replicates as a cancerous cell. In other words, the intelligence of the cell resides in the cell membrane, not in the nucleus. The membrane tells the nucleus what to do. Quite literally, the "brain" is in the cell membrane or the external environment; the nucleus is just the reproductive organ. (How often do human beings confuse their brains and their genitals?)

The pericellular matrix, also called the *glycocalyx,* surrounds the cells of both multicellular and unicellular organisms. In multicellular life-forms, it is used to distinguish between the organisms' own cells, including sick cells within the organism, invading cells, and those transplanted by the knife of the surgeon. It triggers the immune response that kills sick and alien cells. Antirejection drugs are used to suppress this reaction when tissue is transplanted.

The glycocalyx is also found around the cells of epithelial tissue (skin and mucosa) in the higher animals, and in other cells as well. It looks like a fuzzy coating under the microscope, but feels to the touch like the slimy side of a fish. That's because fish skin is coated with a glycocalyx of epithelial cells.

The polysaccharides that compose the glycocalyx are *polymers* (chains of sugar molecules one molecule wide). They are manufactured at the surface of the cell. The glycocalyx not only serves protective and communicative functions but also possesses adhesive properties. We can see how it could have evolved into polymers surrounding groups of cells cloned from the same original to produce something like sea slime.

Going a step further, the slime found on rocks in shallow water is also composed of polymers. This is probably where the first living cells originated and lived, so the glycocalyx may be older than life itself and the "manufacture" of polymers by cells developed from and mimics the way these polymers were first produced on inanimate surfaces.

THE EXTRACELLULAR MATRIX

The first multicellular organisms were created when these clones threw out a line of protective cells to form an external membrane, internalizing a bit of the Great Mother Ocean, creating a compartment to surround and protect themselves. This space between the external membrane and the internal cells is the extracellular matrix, and the materials that are found within it are polysaccharides similar to those in the pericellular matrix, which also possess a protective, communicative, and adhesive function, plus the mineral colloids and electrolytes mentioned below that combine with the water to form a liquid-crystalline gel. The fluid alone is called the *interstitial fluid* while the polymers and fibers are called the *ground substance.* The ECM constitutes about 27.5 percent of the volume of the human body. Although the function of the ECM was largely unknown and ignored until recently, it is not possible to imagine that one-quarter of the human body has no important physiological purpose.

Use of the word *matrix,* instead of *ECM* or *extracellular matrix,* represents more of a "popular science voice" than the other terms, which are more technical.

The fluids inside the cells are called *intracellular,* while all those outside the cells are known as *extracellular fluid* (ECF). The latter are divided into four major divisions: the blood plasma, lymph, cerebrospinal fluid (CSF), and the interstitial fluids in the matrix.

Evolution of the ECM

The first self-enclosed organisms would have been something like a colony of genetically identical cells (a clone) living in a little hole on the seafloor, sending out and surrounded by a mess of polymers, creating what we would call sea slime. The polymers then sent out a signal to some of the cells: migrate to where there are no polymers, that is, to the periphery. This formed the external membranes around the group of cells. This tendency to migrate to where there are no polymers—a "bald spot" in the matrix, so to speak—is still characteristic of cells in the matrix of higher life-forms. It is a method for self-healing and protection.

One would think that the external membrane surrounding the

matrix would have developed first in the course of evolution; the polymers second. However, the reverse is true. Because signals from the polymers control the cells, the latter can't really do anything without the signals: so the polymers existed before the external membrane. The creation of this protective membrane was an evolutionary jump. The evolution of ECM proteins was "key in the transition to multicellularity," and was followed by additional "development of novel protein architectures" (Hynes and Naba 2011), that is to say, tissues and organs. We see, therefore, that the matrix is not only the "brains" of the cell, but the driving force in evolution.

Structure of the ECM

The archaic term for the polymers of the matrix is *polysaccharide.* This is the word used by most herbalists and nutritionists, who are thinking of the slurry of mixed polysaccharides found in an herb or food. The modern technical term is *glycosaminoglycan* (GAG), used in a technical discussion about the anatomy of the matrix. These polysaccharides or GAGs are joined by molecules (called *protein linkers*) to protein "backbones" that form feather-like structures called *proteoglycans* (PGs). These feathery structures are not just thrown together into a tangle, like spaghetti noodles, but highly articulated to fold in or out. They are highly sensitive to water content, folding in if there is less hydration or folding out if there is more. They form organized structural units called *matrisomes* ("matrix-bodies").

In mammals, the basic matrisome is composed of about three hundred proteoglycans, as well as large numbers of enzymes, growth factors, and other proteins associated with the matrix. These constituents contribute to the building, maintenance, and remodeling of the matrix, as well as binding the matrix to the cells. The matrisomes provide inputs into the cells that control the survival, proliferation, shape, polarity, and movement of cells (Hynes and Naba 2011).

The glycosaminoglycans are polymers hundreds or thousands of molecules long (no two are identical), that form the proteoglycans and matrisomes. In addition, there are also short polymers composed of various molecules. Unlike the GAGs, they are not composed largely of sugars and proteins, or organic molecules, but of minerals and trace elements necessary for the onward march of life. They form a stable structure with water that is not susceptible to chemical changes when the matrix contents are in a normal life-sustaining mix. This structure is called a *colloid,* the equilibrium is called the *colloidal state,* and the aggregate of many together in water form a *colloidal solution.* Colloids

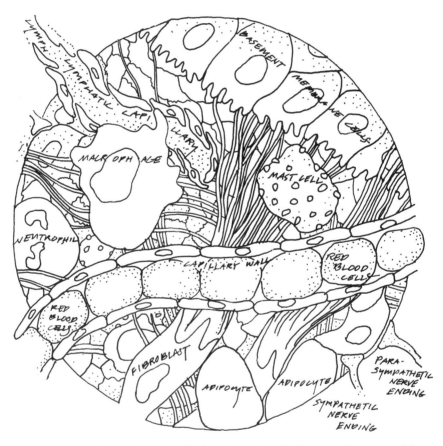

An artistic rendering of the ECM by the author. "Mere visualization of the ECM has been problematic" (Dongari-Bagtzoglou 2008, 201). I hope this illustration provides visual context as you navigate your way through the extracellular matrix.

can form chemical bonds with particles but tend to keep their structural integrity. In this way, they provide the essential and trace elements used by the cells (mostly by the enzymes). They contain both water- and oil-soluble molecules, so they can interact with all the fluids and departments of the living organism. A colloidal solution forms a gel-like or liquid-crystalline material in which the cells, GAGs, proteoglycans, and matrisomes are suspended. The word *colloid* means "glue-like" (Pollack 2001, 2015).

Electrical Charge of the ECM

The matrix polymers, the colloidal polymers, and the larger fibers that eventually evolved to give the organism more structure, carry an overall negative charge. The cell surface has a positive charge. These charges remain stable until some stimulation enters the picture. Then, there is a change in what is called the *electric potential charge,* or the electrical energy in a storage state. This discharge constitutes a signal that controls the messaging in the matrix, moving messages from the surface membrane to the interior—which acts as a single, whole entity—eventually reaching the cells. Through this means, the polymers command the cells when to eat and eliminate, migrate, and procreate. This mechanism was called the *ground regulatory system* by its discoverer, Alfred Pischinger.

Where the potential energy of the surface is minimal in its charge, the surface of the body dips into a saddle-like valley. These small dips can be influenced by even slight stimulation, which, traveling through the matrix, can have profound effects elsewhere. This is the basis of acupuncture points (see Heine's contributions to Pischinger 1991 and Pischinger 2007).

Within the liquid-crystalline "water" of the matrix, there are also *electrolytes,* or single molecules composed of a positively charged ion (*cation*) and one that is negatively charged (*anion*). These have a strong influence on the liquids, particles, and membranes, contributing to the density, charge, and permeability of solutions and solids. The minerals of the colloids and electrolytes are similar in composition to that of the seawater when life originated 4.5 billion years ago, though they are more dilute—about 9 percent, compared with 32 percent.

The Role of Pressure between the ECM and the Blood

In amphibians, the blood and lymph and their carrier tubes are not yet differentiated, so the circulating substance is called *hemolymph*. In higher animals, the blood and lymph are separated and the CSF also appears. The development of the nervous system resulted in the production of CSF, which circulates along the nerves and fills the cavities around nerves compacted in the brain. The choroid plexus, a "sieve" in the brain, separates the CSF out of the blood so that it does not contain red and white blood cells, or blood proteins, but only the refined nutrient, oxygen, and electrolyte mix necessary to maintain the nerves in their active state. In a similar fashion, the serum of the blood is pressed out into the ECM to create the interstitial fluid.

The pressure in the capillary bed is high, forcing the contents into the matrix unless there are high sodium levels, which cause pressure back against the capillary bed, resulting in high blood pressure. Salt collects water, so an excess of water and its contents increases the effect. The pressure in the matrix is greater than that in lymphatic capillaries, so the little gaps or doors in them are pushed open and cause drainage through that system, which empties into the bloodstream just before the heart. A similar process occurs in the venules—the beginning of the venous system on the far side of the capillary bed. Pressure pushes carbon dioxide, water, and ions into the venules, but these substances have to be small because the entrances into the venules are smaller than the gaps in the lymphatic capillaries.

Blood capillaries, tissue membranes, and lymphatic capillaries mark the boundaries of the matrix. These tissue membranes consist of the *basement membrane* and the *interstitium*. The former supports the epithelium of the cells of the skin, mucosa, and serous membranes, while the latter surrounds various organs. The interstitium is an extensive and contiguous extension of the matrix situated between the basement membrane and body organs, including the muscles, circulatory system, and lymphatic vessels. It drains into the veins and lymphatic vessels. It receives its name because it is filled with interstitial fluids, like the rest of the matrix. It saturates the connective tissue or matrix fibers to cause changes in flexibility and shape—also, of course, transmitting matrix signals—all of which control and form the behavior of organs and vessels on the vegetative level of the *parenchyma,* or tissue.

Generation and Regeneration of the Matrix

The matrix polymers are generated by cells—in higher organisms, by specially evolved cells called *fibroblasts.* These eventually also generated connective tissue fibers and finally they evolved and differentiated into cells called *chondroblasts, tenocytes,* and *osteoblasts* that lay down the cartilage, tendon and ligament, and bone, respectively.

Fibroblasts form an important pair with *macrophages,* one of the five basic immune system cells. These two cells control in large measure the generation and removal of the polymers and fibers of the ground substance as it develops and deteriorates. For health to exist, the balance between the generation and removal of proteins in particular must be maintained within narrow parameters. The fibroblasts generate the original tissue, as well as the replacement parts, while macrophages "eat up" and remove the old, worn-out parts. The latter usually arrive in the matrix from the bloodstream, where they modify from *monocytes* (primitive immune cells) into full-fledged macrophages (Olczyk, Mencner, and Komosinska-Vassev 2014; see also chapter 4 in this book).

Regulation of the ECM via the Ground Regulatory System

In their entirety, these mechanisms of communication, the electrical potential charge, binding and growth factors, and fibroblasts and macrophages, as a sum total, constitute the ground regulatory system (GRS), whether in jellyfish or human beings.

ả♥ Mechanical Regulation

There are some additional forms of communication and control of a purely mechanical nature that occur within the matrix. The spaces between the polymers only allow passage of particles under a designated size. In addition, the stiffness, shapes, and orientations of the polymers, fibers, and ligands (binders) influence the behavior of local areas and organs in the body. Indeed, it may be that the deformation of the matrix caused intensifications of function in local areas that led to the development of the organs in the first place. As we will see in chapter 5, the cellular level of function of the organs is controlled by the matrix, including development and ongoing functionality, through the GRS, nerves, circulation, hormones, colloids, and electrolytes that control their operation.

ả♥ Nervous and Endocrine System Regulation

In higher organisms the ECM is intimately tied into the higher regulatory systems—nerves and the endocrine system. Hormones have to move through the matrix to get to their bonding sites in the cells. The cerebrospinal fluid (CFS) eventually dumps out into—where?—the matrix. Thus, the nerves are also tied into the ECM. Of course, matrix polymers cannot "understand" the more sophisticated signaling of the hormones and nerves, but they are sensitive to changes in the levels of hormones and CSF components, since these are causing changes in the makeup of the matrix. In other words, the cellular level of the organism is adapting to changes imposed on it by the higher organism. This means that the matrix is in touch with *everything* going on *everywhere* on the vegetative, vital, or cellular level.

The central nervous system (CNS) gives us the sense of individuality that we as human beings possess, but on the cellular level, we are a mindless vegetable and there is no individualization at all. The two systems (ECM and CNS) are not completely separated, as is often taught, but interconnect and are able to communicate chemically through the fact that all nerve endings terminate in the matrix. This begins a justification of the work of biologists such as Bruce Lipton, who advocate a more intimate relationship between the conscious level and the biological.

SCIENTIFIC JUSTIFICATION OF HOLISTIC MEDICINE

The discovery of the GRS was the fundamental breakthrough in the understanding of the matrix because it demonstrated that it was not just a space filled with water and fluff, but rather an "intelligent" system that controlled the cells and unified them into a single being. The matrix, wrote Pischinger:

> permeates the extracellular spaces of the entire organism, reaches every cell, and always reacts as a unit. (Pischinger 1991, 19; Pischinger 2007, 8)

This has tremendous implications. The first of them is that the organism operates on the cellular level as a *whole* and that the premise of holistic medicine—to treat the organism as a whole, united in operation and intelligence—is fully justified. The reverse is also true: reductionism—seeking meaning in the smallest particle—is not justified as a model for how biological systems work. It is justified simply as a method for understanding the components of the whole, not for comprehending the functions of the whole as a single unit.

From the simplest cell in the ocean to the more complicated animal, the organism and its environment are intimately linked, the whole presiding over smaller subunits or wholes, until we reach the particles, which are either commanded to a purpose by the greater organism or are elements of chaos operating on their own.

Pischinger was a holistic doctor and researcher and was fully conscious of the fact that he had demonstrated the mechanism that makes the body a physiological whole and that provided the scientific justification for holistic medicine.

The matrix operates on the cellular level. This is the basic level on which a plant operates, so it has also been called the "vegetative" level, even in the animal organism. It would seem to be completely restricted in regulatory control and function to this level. Yet, because the nerves find their end in the matrix, there is an influence both "downward" from the higher systems (neuroendocrine) and "upward" from the matrix. This explains psycho-immunology and psychosomatic illness.

> Since the extracellular matrix is connected to the endocrine gland system via the capillaries, and to the central nervous system via the peripheral vegetative nerve endings with their blind endings in the extracellular matrix, and both systems are connected to each other in the brain stem, superior regulatory centers can be influenced by the extracellular matrix. (Pischinger 1991, 20)

As the holy grail of medical and biological reductionism, the cell theory is shown by these discoveries to be an illusion. The cell is not the "ultimate unit" of biological life, in a functional sense, but is only a part of the primal functional unit, which Pischinger denominated the capillary-matrix-cell. We cannot speak of the cell as an individual: all cells are bound together into a communication network.

ORGAN INDEPENDENCE

Although the matrix unifies the organism into a whole, there are, at the same time, differences from one compartment or organ to another. Each organ is surrounded by a serous membrane that separates it in some measure from the matrix as a whole. Even bundles of muscles are grouped into compartments separated by serous membranes, and the same is true for the larger blood vessels and nerves, which travel together in bundles to their various destinations.

The matrix of each organ in a multicellular animal develops with the organ, both before and after birth, and there is a constant interplay between matrix and organ. This means that there are unique neuro-endocrine and neuropsychological connections with every organ. This is an ancient idea in natural and alternative medicine, seen in the old idea of the zodiacal man in astrology, in which the signs are linked to the organs, then emotions and health functions. This explains why many herbs have both a specific emotional and biological activity. Laypeople, medical doctors, and complementary and alternative medicine practitioners all adhere to the idea of organ-specific strengths and weaknesses.

Not only does the local matrix regulate the organ it surrounds, but it also selects the materials that will be pulled into the space. Even the type of cells drawn in from the circulation can differ from tissue to tissue, or organ to organ, due to the differing composition of the matrix in each compartment. The fates of these incoming cells, their differentiation, and their applications are also modified by the local matrix.

The matrix then controls the differentiation into different cell types of these new inhabitants of the matrix and their behavior and function, as well as controlling the distribution of the materials entering the matrix. It turns out that all cells are inherently epigenetic. This is because the ECM "has a significant effect on determining the genetic expressivity of a cell" (Pischinger 1991, 14). This also shows us that evolution is not Darwinian; that is to say, it is not driven by random mutations in genetic material, but by the environment, which produces adaptive effects within the cells.

All of these compartments are full of ground substance (polymers, colloids, fibers) and are still in contact with each other, though they are also separated by serous membranes. The matrix signals communicate throughout, crossing the membranes, but there is some autonomy from structure to structure and region to region and the polymer and collagen makeup can be very different. In addition, new regulatory methods evolved, first the endocrine system (chemicals or hormones diffusing through the matrix) and then the nervous system (electrical signaling along neuron cells and tracts).

THE MATRIX IS THE ORIGINAL ORGAN/SYSTEM

Another implication of Pischinger's research is that the matrix is the primal or original organ/system of the body. Like any organ, it possesses a location: everywhere in the body that lies between the cells, the capillary bed, and the lymphatic capillaries. Like any organ or system, it possesses a function: protecting, controlling, unifying, and regulating cell life. Because it was the first structure generated by multicellular organisms, we must look on it as the first organ system of all life-forms. This means that it is therapeutically essential because it determines the environment and conditions of cellular life. Thus, it is a primary as well as primal organ system, and yet, it is almost completely ignored in modern biomedical therapy. Instead, it is actively attacked by modern drugs, which bypass the matrix, ignore the GRS, and thereby weaken self-regulation and self-cure within the organism.

The second organ system in the animal economy almost immediately makes its appearance on the stage of life. The fibers that are generated in the matrix by the fibroblasts are the first evidences of the connective tissue system. Fibroblasts are the primal connective tissue cell, from which are developed all the other connective tissue cells (chondroblasts, tenocytes, and osteoblasts).

Although the matrix is largely ignored in modern biomedicine, it is, conversely, the basis of treatment in virtually all systems of ancient, traditional, indigenous, complimentary, and alternative forms of medicine. These methods are based on the treatment of the underlying condition of "humors" (fluids) or "energies" in the organism. While biomedicine ignores the matrix and bypasses it therapeutically by directing drugs to receptors on the cell membrane, holistic and natural forms of medicine act on the whole organism through this primal organ system. When we fully understand the ECM, we at last will be able to explain the basis of many holistic therapies, including acupuncture points and meridians, massage, cupping, the manipulative arts, and herbalism. The implications of the discovery of the GRS and the ECM are vast and revolutionary.

DEATH OF THE CELL THEORY

In 1858, Rudolf Virchow purposed that disease be defined as a disturbance in the structure of the individual cell. Each cell was viewed as an "elemental organism" that took care of itself within a community of self-regulating cells, forming altogether the greater organism. As Virchow explained:

> The chief point in this application of histology to pathology is to obtain a recognition of the fact that the cell is really the ultimate morphological element in which there is any manifestation of life, and that we must not transfer the seat of real action to any point beyond the cell. (Virchow 1971, 29)

This is known as the cell theory. Biology has been based on it, and still largely is today, yet it has been overthrown by the discovery of the GRS, which is not a *theory* but a *fact*.

The primitive view of Virchow was easy to understand—even intuitive—since the individual cell superficially resembles the individual human in society. Unfortunately, it turns out to be completely incorrect. Not only has a primary paradigm of modern medicine, the cell theory, been overturned, but it has also been shown to be what it actually is: an ideation characteristic of the linear, cause-and-effect, reductionist thinking typical of Western science in the past three and a half centuries. It is not inherently an accurate picture of how the natural world works as a whole community, inside and outside the organism. It is a projection of human individualism onto a biological level in which there is no individualism whatsoever.

This overthrows not only the conceptual foundation of modern science and medicine itself but also conventional therapeutic models and practices. "The entire therapeutic system of academic medicine is affected by this linearity in medical thought," writes Pischinger.

> In attempting to cling to the simplistic viewpoint of cause-and-effect relationships, one has no choice but to separate the acute event from its intermeshed biological associations, call it a syndrome, and treat it as if it were an isolated event. (Pischinger 2007, 3)

The cell theory implies therapy based on an isolated molecule, a drug, which will find a suitable cell receptor in the membrane of the cell, to which it can attach and then influence. This theory dominates teaching, clinical trials, and practice, but it does not conform to the way the body actually operates.

> Reality is replaced by models. (Pischinger 2007, 3)

Medical treatment directed to the molecular lesion in the cell bypasses the GRS and is therefore inherently disruptive of the self-regulation of the life-form. By weakening the primary organizational force within the organism, drug therapy is therefore ultimately destructive rather than healing. What we call the side effects of drugs are minimized, whereas they are in fact symptoms indicating the presence of a destructive process grinding down the resistance of the organism. The whole of modern biomedicine is therefore founded on a misconception and is not health promoting but ultimately disease promoting.

The success of modern biomedicine is primarily due to changes in public health and to the suppression of acute diseases by simple methods that work in almost everyone (e.g., antibiotics, cortisol). But increasingly, modern people are being afflicted by mysterious diseases that cannot be explained by the established medical model. Examples include autism (one child in twenty-seven in one community), immunological diseases, all sorts of cancers, sensitivities to electricity and other invisible frequencies, Lyme disease and its numerous coinfections, childhood cancers, and the exploding rates of diabetes. More than thirty years ago, Pischinger observed that the biomedical model "is seldom successful with the increasingly prevalent chronic diseases and tumors." On the other hand, the Vienna school claimed success in the treatment of chronic illnesses over more than four generations (Pischinger 1991).

About 1950, notes Arthur Firstenberg, medicine became profoundly corrupted by modern industry (Firstenberg 2016). Medicine could either acknowledge that tens of thousands of unexamined chemical toxins and electrical influences new to the environment had unknown or questionable health effects, or it could ignore them in order to enable modern corporate industry. Medicine really had no choice: it could not object to the juggernaut of the modern economy. From this time forward, medicine became more aggressive in asserting its opinions and suppressing its opponents.

If Pischinger's scientific research is valid, then why is it not better known? Pischinger only addresses the conceptual problems, not the juggernaut of modern industry. He explains that it is because linear, cause-and-effect, reductionist thinking is easier to understand, despite the wholesale divorce from the reality of biology entailed by this approach. Virchow's "more easily comprehended concept of 'cells'" fit the reductionist theory prevalent in Western science, which emphasized "the smallest building blocks of an organism" (Pischinger 2007, 4).

In the last twenty years, the understanding of the complexity and depth of communication and regulation within the organism, as well as within plant communities—even among unrelated species—has grown by leaps and bounds. It is increasingly clear that life is highly organized, self-regulating, and complex, and that our simplistic cell theory and drug therapeutics are medieval in conception and destructiveness.

Why are we still using primitive medical, agricultural, and biological premises that are damaging our planet? Habit, self-indulgence, and the profit motive are driving the continuing use of these destructive methods.

Science is subject to the inertia of scientists. The atomic physicist Max Planck made a comment that is widely quoted (in various paraphrases):

Science advances one funeral at a time.

The overthrow of the cell theory returns us to the ancient "humoral" approach found in various forms in nearly all systems of traditional medicine. It also reopens the debate on the importance of the individual bacterium or virus as a causative agent of disease versus the *terrain* or environment in which the microorganism travels and multiplies. The introduction of a germ does not necessarily mean that it will flourish and reproduce; this depends in part on the environment in which it finds itself. Research shows that both healthy and unhealthy populations generally maintain a similar internal biota, with the exception of certain dangerous epidemic disease organisms that strike down everyone (Yang 2012).

Pischinger's discoveries return us to the era in medicine when the local terrain and the constitution of the individual were considered as important or more important than local disease and the presence of microorganisms. His work justifies the approach of herbalism, homeopathy, and other forms of natural medicine that direct treatment toward the individual as a whole, the internal terrain, the constitution, or the major processes and functions, organs and systems, rather than bacteria, isolated cell receptor sites, and microscopic changes. It also justifies massage, acupuncture, cupping, and other forms of local treatment that act on humoral and/or energetic imbalances in local areas of the matrix. It does not, of course, completely abrogate the germ theory, the applications of which, through public health and antibiotics, have revolutionized life on Earth. But there is a need for a correct perspective, not an absolutist dogma.

The Germ Theory

The cell theory was reinforced by the germ theory, which is associated with the name of Louis Pasteur (1822–1895). He taught that in health the interior of the organism was essentially sterile and that disease was caused by the introduction of microbes. His theory left no room for the idea that some form of susceptibility in the organism invited in bacteria. The germ theory helped further crush humoralism because the microbe, like the cell, was seen as the ultimate basis of pathology. The environment of both the cell and the germ seemed unimportant.

One of the opponents of Pasteur was Antoine Béchamp (1816–1908). He claimed that disease arose due to a susceptibility in the environment of the body, allowing the bacteria to proliferate. Béchamp called the internal environment of the organism, whether healthy or unhealthy, the *terrain*. Unfortunately, this rather sensible idea was tied to his theory that bacterial cells evolved from a prebacterial state to a full-fledged bacterium under the influence of the disturbed terrain. This aspect of the theory must be relegated to the dustbin of history. Modern research on the microbiome shows that both the healthy and the sick host the same basic bacteria, not in a nascent but in a fully developed state, awaiting changes in the environment (terrain) to be released (Yang 2012).

Pasteur was correct in many regards, but we now know that the body is not a sterile medium waiting for infection by an external bacterium but rather a complex microbiome full of friendly and unfriendly microbes. The microbiome can change a friendly bacterium to an unfriendly one, and back and forth. The introduction and proliferation of damaging microbes certainly cause disease, whether it be E. coli, malaria, or Lyme disease, but the microbiome and the terrain cannot be entirely ignored. Susceptibility can cause or magnify the effect of microbes. The body attempts to maintain a steady balance that controls microbial proliferation. The homeostatic mechanism is always at work to help maintain the internal environment of the organism in a state where microbes cannot unduly multiply. However, stress knocks the organism off-balance and it becomes susceptible.

Unfortunately, the simplistic view of Virchow and Pasteur triumphed and modern medicine was birthed. The germ theory caused a huge leap forward in public health because the germs leading to infectious diseases were isolated and removed from the external environment. Although the cell theory can now be proved to be incorrect altogether and the germ theory needs to be modified, modern biomedicine continues to act (at least as far as therapy is concerned) as if nothing fundamental had shifted.

Recantations?

It is often stated in complementary and alternative medicine that late in life Virchow recanted his view, making the following statement:

> If I could live my life over again, I would devote it to proving that germs seek their natural habitat—diseased tissue—rather than being the cause of the diseased tissue, in the way that mosquitoes seek the stagnant water, but do not cause the pool to become stagnant.

Strangely, this is not a recantation of the work of Virchow, but of Pasteur! Since this statement is often quoted in alternative medical literature, I tracked it down to its original source, *The Finer Forces of Nature in Diagnosis and Therapy* by Dr. George S. White (1939, 139). White says he had the above statement from an unnamed "pupil of Adolph Virchow" (*sic*).

Much as we would like to believe that Virchow saw the error of his ways late in life, hearsay cannot be considered a credible source, and getting Virchow's name wrong makes it clear that White did not carefully document whatever it was he heard from whomever it was who made the statement—if the statement was made at all.

It is also said that Pasteur recanted his position on his deathbed. Hans Selye, the famous physiologist, gives an account of this in *The Stress of Life* (1956). Dr. Rénon, who was taking care of Pasteur, reported that the old man said, *"Bernard avait raison. Le germe n'est rien, c'est le terrain est tout"* ("Bernard was right. The germ is nothing, the terrain is everything" or "The seed is nothing, the soil is everything").

This statement was not made up by Selye; it appears in many French medical texts, to judge from my survey of the internet. However, the wording of the recantation refers to the terminology of Béchamp, rather than that of Claude Bernard (1813–1878), one of the founders of modern physiology. The term *terrain* is characteristic of the former, while Bernard used the term *milieu intérieur.* Therefore, this statement, too, seems somewhat questionable.

Alternative practitioners have hung their hopes on the idea that the founders of biomedicine recanted their theories late in life. We need no longer entertain these hopes because modern research has simply proved these positions to be naïve and untenable. There was absolutely no way that scientists in 1858 could have understood the inner workings of the organism with their primitive tools. Sadly, the crude "scientific" theories (and they were only theories) generated at this time are still to this day the foundation of biology and medicine.

Resistance to the Cell Theory

Although the cell theory triumphed for a century and a half, a small minority of physicians and scientists refused to abandon the humoral model. The only major center of serious scientific resistance within the medical profession was at the medical school of the University of Vienna. Opposition began with Virchow's contemporaries.

Carl von Rokitansky, the leading voice at the University of Vienna, observed that pathological changes are accompanied by modifications in circulation. He therefore objected to considering the cell the exclusive determinant of health. The cell was dependent on the capillary blood flow (also the lymphatic drainage, it would turn out), which conditioned its environment. Rokitansky's reputation was great enough that a compromise of sorts was reached in German medicine, preserving a healthy respect for the circulation.

In *Traditional Western Herbalism and Pulse Evaluation* (Wood, Bonaldo, and Light 2016), I cited the work of Dr. Irvin Korr (1997), an osteopath who demonstrated that pathological expressions in the organism are accompanied by circulatory changes unique to each case (not each disease name). The circulation is controlled by the sympathetic nervous system, which contracts the peripheral arterioles that control the amount of blood flowing into an area. The parasympathetic nervous system does not have a direct influence. Any particular disease state is characterized by changes in circulation that bring blood to or keep blood from an area. Each presentation is unique: changes in local sympathetic tone do not conform to artificially imposed diagnostic categories but are unique to each pathological presentation. Korr's work was inclusive, exhaustive, and gathered from numerous sources.

> The evidence is in four categories: a) symptomatology and pathophysiology; b) chronic experimental stimulation; c) interruption or reduction of sympathetic activity; and d) morphological changes in ganglia and other sympathetic components. (Korr 1997, 70)

Traditional osteopathy influences pathology through two major pathways—the muscular and skeletal system and the circulation. Korr emphasized the association of the sympathetic somatic muscles and their treatment.

> In approaching the role of the sympathetic nervous system (SNS) in disease, it is important to have a good perspective of its function in normal life. W. R. Hess emphasized its "ergotropic" function, that of adjusting circulation, metabolism and visceral activity according to musculoskeletal, postural and environmental demand. These adjustments include changes in cardiac output, distribution of blood flow by regulation of peripheral resistance, heat dissipation and release of peripheral resistance, heat dissipation and release of stored metabolites. These adjustments are of systemic nature, yet they have a high degree of localization according to the site and amount of muscular activity. (Korr 1997, 70)

The importance of the "circulation" was widely assumed and used in both alternative and conventional medicine in the nineteenth and early twentieth centuries. We observe it extensively in both major schools of botanical medicine originating in America: physiomedicalism and eclecticism. "Equalize the circulation" was a byword of this era. As recently as 1930, conventional medical books would title a chapter "Circulation," not "Cardiovascular System."

Rokitansky's model is still recognized in German medicine today. I once attended a lecture where the herbalist Simon Mills placed the conception of Gingko against this background. He explained that in Germany the idea that disease is accompanied by circulatory change is widely acknowledged and that this led to the development of a drug specific for the circulation—Gingko.

This is the correct way to explain the properties of a medicinal plant. The background of the medical or folkloric suppositions in which it came to prominence need to be comprehended in order to understand these uses. Without cultural context, we often cannot fully appreciate the application or action of an herb. History and folk tradition are as important as pharmacology because they establish the context in which an idea arose.

It should be remarked that Rokitansky's argument was quite different from Korr's. Rokitansky believed that the circulation was modified by plaque on the vessel linings caused by clotting of the blood. This was supposedly disproven by Virchow, who showed that the blood clots were covered over by epithelium and therefore had no direct effect on vascular health. Today, we know that the blood carries what are called endothelial progenitor cells that alight on a recently deposited clot or thrombus and generate an epithelial covering. The epithelium grows over the clots to prevent them from breaking off and causing strokes. These narrowings change the circulation, so in fact Rokitansky was correct. Korr adhered to a simpler model, which is also correct: sympathetic tensions in the arterioles change circulation.

An additional repercussion of this debate was that cardiovascular disease came to be attributed to cholesterol deposition, based on Virchow's theory, whereas Rokitansky's suggests that it is a slowdown in the production of endothelial progenitor cells that causes stroke and heart attack. This occurs with aging, stress, steroid medication, and kidney disease, all of which are associated with greatly increased dangers of cardiovascular disease (Kendrick 2013).

In the generation following Rokitansky, the opposition of the Vienna school to the germ theory was carried forward by Hans Eppinger Jr. (1879–1946), a professor of internal medicine at the university before the Second World War. Eppinger developed Rokitansky's proposals further, maintaining that healthy circulation produced a suitable environment for every cell. He called the material making up this environment the *ground substance.*

Unfortunately, today Eppinger is best remembered as one of the Nazi "monster doctors" involved in horrible experiments carried out at Dachau, a Nazi concentration camp that was committed primarily to torture rather than genocide. When the Nuremberg trials started, he committed suicide, leaving funds of unknown origin in a Swiss bank account. If he were not credited with the idea of the ground substance by Pischinger, I certainly would not have known that he belonged in the "chain of transmission" that led to the discovery of the GRS and the overturning of the cell theory. I doubt this information would show up anywhere near the top of the references to Eppinger on Google.

The importance of the circulation was diminished from 1930 onward, but the Vienna school continued in their obstinacy, developing therapeutic models for the chronic illnesses that biomedicine was increasingly ignoring as its concept of disease became increasingly narrow. Part of this was due to the success of modern biomedicine and public health, but there was the additional reason pointed out by Firstenberg: medicine had to become more arrogant than it had ever been before to protect industry. From 1950 onward, medicine was a part of the medical-industrial complex and was actively engaged in ignoring evidence. It was increasingly founded on dogmatic assertions that are unproven or simply wrong.

For my generation of practitioners, this was not theoretical. In 1956, V. E. Irons was brought to trial for asserting that white bread was not as healthy as whole wheat bread. Since he was obviously in the wrong (thought the judge) and it was against the law to oppose established facts important to the generation of money and the reputation of modern medicine, he was offered the opportunity of recanting his claim in exchange for a suspended sentence rather than serving six months in prison. He chose the latter. In 1983, the Amish farmer and herbalist Solomon Wickey was brought to trial for practicing medicine without a license. Dr. John Christopher was so hounded that he could only teach, not practice. In 1985, Dr. Carl Reich lost his medical license for advocating calcium supplementation. When I began to work at the herb store in 1982, we daily feared arrest by the Board of Medical Practice, and one of our friends, a naturopath licensed in Washington State but practicing in Minnesota, was arrested as late as 1997. Those of us who "practiced medicine without a license" in those years will never forget them.

Another graduate of the University of Vienna medical school who advocated comparatively holistic ideas was Hans Selye (1907–1982), who developed the ideas of stress and adaptation, which are so important for understanding the function of the adrenals and immune system in maintaining homeostasis. We will take his work up in the appendix.

Another early advocate of the importance of the ECM in physiology, pathology, and therapy was Marguerite Maury. Educated as a nurse in Vienna at a time when it was impossible for a woman to receive a doctorate in medicine there, she later immigrated to France, where she became a medical doctor and single-handedly resuscitated the moribund practice of aromatherapy. Although she quoted French research, it is possible she too was influenced by the Viennese impulse. Her findings will be discussed more in chapter 6, "The In-Mix-Out of the Matrix."

RETURN TO HUMORAL MEDICINE

The ECM encompasses or touches upon epithelial cells, the basement membrane, macrophages, fibroblasts, collagen fibers, mast cells, the capillary bed, GAGs, PGs, colloids, electrolytes, and, in the higher animals, nerve endings. Pischinger remarks, "The result is a vast, complex, intermeshed humoral system, whose historical scientific predecessors are to be found in the classical vital juice theory" of the ancient and traditional medical systems developed throughout the world (1991, 20).

Until the appearance of Virchow's cell theory, the universal medical approach was humoralism—the idea that imbalances in the fluids of the body caused ill-health. Hippocrates defined health as the proper *eucrasia* (healthy mixture) of fluids, while disease was defined as a *dyscrasia* (dysfunctional mixture). Consequently, moving, cleansing, purging, or tonifying the humors through the use of massage, cupping, bleeding, moxibustion, acupuncture, bone setting, dieting, and herbal treatment was standard protocol. These ideas and practices concur both in ancient Greece and virtually every corner of the world. The work of Pischinger returns medicine to the humoral model, to the Great Mother Ocean, to timeless, sensible treatment.

When physiological research began in the West, medicine was still based on humoralism. The progenitor of modern histology, Dr. Marie François Xavier Bichat (1771–1802; yes, he died at age thirty-one) designated the space around the cells as the *lacunary system,* filled with *lacunary fluid.* Here is a sympathetic description of Bichat's idea:

> These parenchymatous lymph spaces cannot be considered as lymph capillaries, because they are not invested with the characteristic epithelioid lining, which forms the wall of the latter. They represent a diffuse system of lacunae, interstitial to the cells of the various tissues, which, according to Bichat's doctrine, is generally regarded as the origin of the vascular lymphatic system, i.e., of that provided with characteristic walls. In many invertebrates the lacunar system,

which has no proper wall, is the only one that co-exists with the blood vascular system; so that we may logically regard the lymphatic vascular system as a perfecting, a canalization or successive centralizing of the primary lacunar or interstitial system. (Luciani 1911, 37)

This is a beautiful account of the transformation from the free-fluid environment of the matrix into the channel-controlled drainage of the lymphatic system. We can see that Luciani is grasping at terms and concepts to describe the matrix because there really were no terms for it at the time. Eventually, the term *lacunary system* came to be applied in conventional biology only to amphibians and ancient creatures that have a general, undifferentiated blood-lymph-interstitial fluid bathing the internal spaces. Both blood vessels and lymphatic ducts then developed out of this generalized space.

In the invertebrates or animals without backbones, there is not a clear distinction between blood, tissue fluid and lymph, since they all move through the same vascular spaces and body cavities, and are collectively called "haemo-lymph." Invertebrates and lower fishes do not seem to possess lymphatic vessels and they are first encountered in the bony fishes and amphibia. (Groves 2004, 16)

For Maury, the term *lacunary system* presented a different inspiration. She used the term to describe the compartment around the cells, the ECM. It is interesting to see how a holistic thinker/doctor was driven to include the matrix in her writings, even before it "officially existed."

A more elegant term for the internal space between the cells was introduced by Bernard. It was initially ignored by medicine due to the enthusiasm surrounding the appearance of Virchow's cell theory, but Cannon revived it in the 1920s, and it has been adopted by modern medicine and biology: *milieu intérieur*. This phrase appears in several works published by Bernard between 1854 and his death in 1878.

Bernard realized that no matter what the cells were doing, they were dependent on the environment around them. This established the "milieu" in which they lived. Cannon introduced the term *homeostasis* to describe the ongoing balance that must be maintained within parameters in the space around the cells in order for life to maintain itself. Homeostasis is always slightly fluctuating as the body counters external and internal changes. Interestingly, the pH level in the matrix actually has to change a great deal in order for different biochemical actions to take place within it, so variation in balance is required.

It is believed that Bernard adopted the term *milieu intérieur* from another Parisian cell biologist, Charles Robin, who used the phrase *milieu de l'intérieur* to describe the Hippocratic humors (Gross 1998, 383). Bernard's "internal milieu" therefore directly descended from the ancient humoral model.

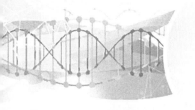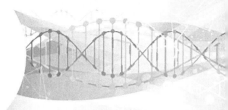

2

What Is Going On in There?
Water, Light, Warmth, Oxidation, Chemistry, and Electricity

Even the mere visualization of the ECM has been problematic.

ANNA DONGARI-BAGTZOGLOU (2008)

One half the sea, one half the flash of lightning.

HERAKLEITOS THE DARK (C. 500 BCE)

The major function of the ECM is to provide an environment for the cells. In this, it needs to keep steady levels of warmth, moisture, structure, and nutrition. Since it is simultaneously a communication system, it also transfers electrical, chemical, and biological substances and messages from area to area. In order to understand how the ECM functions as a whole, we need to understand these major processes.

In holistic medicine, we do not overlook broad natural forces such as warmth, light, water, and electricity in the life of the organism. In fact, we tend to emphasize these grand themes. In conventional medicine and biology, the emphasis is more heavily placed on molecular structure. These two orientations reflect the differences between holism and reductionism. Before going on to the molecular structure of the matrix, we therefore will discuss these grand themes.

THE SPECIAL PROPERTIES OF WATER

Water is the ideal medium for establishing a stable environment for the cells because it possesses a high *specific heat,* a term that refers to the ability of a substance to absorb or release heat without moving into a new phase—from liquid to vapor or solid. Between 32° and 212°F (0° and 100°C), water stays in the same phase—liquid. If water cooled off quickly (like french fries) or heated up quickly (like wax), it could not provide a stable environment for life.

> Water has a much higher specific heat than most substances, a fact of great biologic significance. Body composition is based on solutions and colloidal dispersions that are aqueous. Thus the specific heat of water promotes thermal stability in tissues and the internal environment, which thereby can gain or lose considerable heat without a concomitant change in their temperature. (Ramsey 1982, 143)

This quotation points to a second important property of water: it makes an excellent medium within which the particles and components of life can disperse and become available to cells. This allows for feeding and waste removal. Food travels through fluids—blood plasma, serum, lymph—to arrive at the cell membrane, where it is needed. We should not think of this water, especially in the matrix and the cell, as a lake or pond, but as a gel or "liquid crystal" through which material is transported by electron signals. In the blood and the lymph, substances travel more freely, but here too they are ultimately heavily controlled by regulatory mechanisms. As far as elimination is concerned, the simplest organisms have the same philosophy of garbage removal we have: dump it in the ocean.

Water dissolves minerals carried within it and tries to buffer their charges if they are too positive or negative. H_2O dissociates into hydrogen ions (H+) and hydroxyl molecules (OH−). The hydrogen ions buffer acids formed by metabolism in the cells. An excess of H+ causes a high, alkaline pH level in the fluids; a low amount results in an acid state (pH level below 7.0). Blood is buffered at a strict pH level between 7.35 and 7.45, but it turns out that the pH level of the matrix needs to fluctuate up and down in order for various chemical and biological operations to take place within it (Marunaka 2015).

Salts that are hard and mineralized in the absence of water dissociate into positive and negative ions in water, and in this form, they control the movement, solubility, and activities of water. Sodium chloride attracts water, while sodium sulfate drives it out. Electrolytes consist of a positively charged ion, like sodium, and a negatively charged ion, like chlorine, or an acid, like sulfate ($-SO_2$). There is a mild electrical bond between the positively and negatively charged ions—the cations and anions—while they are dissolved in water, so that each pole is loosely associated with the other. The alkali, or base, and the acid can thus be separated so that each can be used in some chemical reaction in the body. Thus, water not only carries substances but also makes them available (or not) for chemical transformation.

These dissociations of cations and anions like $H+$ or $Na+$ or $Ca++$ from $Cl-$ or $-SO_2$ or $OH-$ set up the potential for electron flow or electricity. As we know, water can conduct electricity. This property too makes water an excellent media for life. The most rapid electrical signaling occurs through the nerves, which are saturated in CSF. A slower signaling method, called piezoelectricity, moves along the connective tissue. On the level of the matrix and the cell, electrical charges remain constant until there is an alteration that provokes a sudden change in charge—like a quantum change. The GRS is the least dynamic but most all-inclusive of the signaling mechanisms of the organism, bringing information to the doorstep of every cell.

Although we have been thinking of water in terms of H_2O, within the living organism the water molecules dissociate into an H_3O+/H_3O_2- complex that carries a mild electrical charge. Since this charge is slightly negative, the structured water helps to transmit the GRS electron signals sent by the polymers of the matrix, which are also negatively charged, to the surface of the cell. This special water forms a crystalline substance that is neither liquid nor solid, leading Gerald Pollack (2015) to describe it as the *fourth phase* of water. This structured water is found in all organisms and is necessary for life to take place; in fact, life began in water exposed to sunlight. In order to discuss this fourth phase or special property of water, we need to understand the special properties of sunlight acting on water and life-forms.

THE SPECIAL PROPERTIES OF SUNLIGHT ON WATER

Gerald Pollack's (2015) research shows that when sunlight hits water (H_2O) on a hydrophilic (water-loving) surface, it splits the water molecule into H_3O_2- and a hydronium ion (H_3O+). Usually, the positively charged hydronium ion is set between two negatively charged H_3O_2 molecules, forming a viscid, alkaline, liquid-crystalline substance that holds a slightly negative overall charge. This forms a "gel" within the intracellular and interstitial fluids.

All the water inside the living organism is composed of this modified water, which Pollack labeled *EZ water*. This means that life began on hydrophilic surfaces where this water was naturally being formed by sunlight. Organisms internalized this kind of water, but proximity to the sun kept renewing the water within them as well. Sunlight still does this to higher life-forms like ourselves because it passes through the peripheral tissues of the body. Put a flashlight up to your hand or fingers in the dark, and the light will shine through; sunlight penetrates through the surface of organic tissue.

Many of the processes of life require the properties of this fourth phase of water. The polymers in the cells and the matrix are saturated with "living" water that hydrates them and contributes to their negative electric charge. It stores energy, which it can also discharge. A steady charge in the environment of the polymers is very important, as well as the discharge of energy. Therefore, EZ water is part of the GRS.

Hydration levels soften or harden the polymers to create different levels of flexibility, hardness, and softness.

The process of making EZ water is similar to that of several important chemical processes in the living cell. For instance, the basic method used by the plant kingdom to make energy from the sun (photosynthesis) is modeled on this conversion, while the conversion in the opposite direction is the basis of animal life. The molecules used for these processes, chlorophyll and hemoglobin, are porphyrins, the molecules that enable movement of electrons in organic and inorganic substances. We will come back to these remarkable substances in a bit.

Although created in a liquid form, fourth-phase water can be both vaporized and precipitated. Rising into the atmosphere, it forms droplets with the hydronium ions in the center and the H_3O_2 ions in the perimeter. This produces an "edge" on the droplet that gives it greater individual cohesion; that is, longer continuity as a droplet. The overall negative charge on the outside of the droplet attracts positively charged energy from the earth, so some lightning discharges upward from the earth into the clouds. This resembles the way charges will flow along the molecular polymers of the saturated matrix, bringing messages to and from the cells. The polymers are negatively charged, but they attract and discharge electricity, like the Earth itself. As the droplets falling from the sky merge together, they again assume the liquid-crystalline form of fourth-phase water. Rainwater, therefore, is fourth-phase water and is more supportive of organic life than the water obtained from plumbing or wells (Pollack 2015).

Holistic EZ Water–Based Treatments

One of my friends was advised by a Vietnamese doctor to "throw water on roof, drink." At the time, we thought it was a rather quaint folk-medical prescription, but now we know that there is a scientific reason for attributing medicinal powers to rainwater and dew: they are water in the fourth phase and are therefore empowered and similar to the water in our bodies.

The alchemists of old called the fluid in the body "dew" because they observed that the biological fluids were slightly more cohesive than normal water. They noted the edge that forms more readily on the drop. They also saw this in the dew on plants and as gathered it as a medicinal substance. Herbalists here will think of Lady's Mantle (*Alchemilla vulgaris*), the plant that maintains the dew in the folds of its leaves longer than any other common plant. Her name comes from the raincoat-like effect of her leaves (like a lady's mantle) and the collection of the dew: *Alchemilla* means the "little alchemist."

Plants absorb dew more slowly, over a longer period of the day, compared with the absorption rate of the groundwater around the roots, demonstrating a significant biological difference. Cohesive water also possesses a lower electrical charge, meaning it is closer to neutral and can interact with alkaline or acid, positively or negatively charged substances and electrolytes.

Dr. Edward Bach originally made his famous flower essences from dew collected from flowers. Later, he made the preparation easier for the layperson: soak the flowers in a bowl of water in sunlight until the flowers lose their healthy appearance. This would, of course, create EZ water. *While we have no scientific proof, it stands to reason that this form of water would extract plant properties differently from ordinary water.* Now, we understand that these practices are significant in biological terms and not just odd, quaint, or "mystical."

A factor in the transmission of light into and through the organism is the availability of the element of silicon. This puts a smooth sheen on the surfaces of connective tissue, including the blood vessels, reducing the production of heat by friction while facilitating the movement of heat and water. This sheen is visible in grasses, which depend on silicon for their structural material. Rudolf Steiner, the Austrian philosopher and founder of anthroposophy, pointed out that plants with thistles and needles are high is silicon, which, from the elemental level (Si_2) to the physical (flint) is the sharpest element. We should be mindful of the need for silicon (homeopathic Silicea) when the hair, eyes, mind, and skin lack sheen. Dull hair and skin lack the reflective qualities of the silicon seen in glass, obsidian, and flint. More importantly, perhaps, silicon conveys light, so it is important in bringing light into the body. Think here of the grasses *Avena* (Oatstraw), *Equisetum* (Horsetail), which is rich in silicon, and sharp-thorned *Dipsacus* (Teasel).

The manufacture of fourth-phase water by sunlight creates energy, and this chemical reaction resembles photosynthesis, by which plants harvest energy from the sun. The production of fourth-phase water follows this formula:

$$\text{sunlight} + \text{hydrophilic surface} + (3)\ H_2O < H_3O_2 - H_3O+$$

Compare this with the formula for photosynthesis:

$$\text{sunlight} + \text{chlorophyll molecule} + (6)\ H_2O + (6)\ CO_2 < C_6H_{12}O_6\ (\text{glucose}) + (6)\ O_2$$

Chlorophyll is made from a ring of porphyrins combined with a magnesium atom. This produces a reactive molecule that absorbs energy from light and transfers it to an electron that leaves the chlorophyll for an electron transport chain that ultimately produces glucose. This is an oxidative process, so the chlorophyll gives up some oxygen as well. This is replaced by oxygen from carbon dioxide and an electron from a molecule of water.

The oxygen made by plants as a waste product long ago saturated the atmosphere, making it 70 percent oxygen. This is taken up by the hemoglobin molecule in the blood of animals, which is identical to the chlorophyll molecule except that it has an iron instead of a magnesium atom in the crucial place in the structure. Both are porphyrins, which may be described briefly as light-sensitive, pigmented, four-cornered molecules. Chlorophyll molecules provide the green color of plants; the iron in hemoglobin provides the red color of oxygenated blood.

Not only did fourth-phase water form a sort of template that living organisms later used to generate energy, Pollack and his fellow researchers also found that charged EZ water is attracted into and moves through a narrow hydrophilic tube, thus anticipating the movement of life fluids—similar to the movement of sap in a tree or blood in a human being (Pollack 2015). Prick your finger and place a thin glass pipette against the drop of blood: it will move up the glass. Even normal water will exploit physical properties to move through a capillary. When the hydrophilic pull of the water to the membrane is higher than the pull between the water molecules, the water is pulled along by the capillaries (Rattle et al. 2013).

It should be evident that blood is not moved by the heart alone, but also by a complimentary set of activities in the arteries and the tiny hydrophilic capillaries that hungrily draw in the blood serum and its contents. Doppler imaging shows that blood flows through the capillaries of the fetus before the heart is formed (Marinelli et al., 1995).

Even color is significant in the great symphony of life. Sunlight splits into the color spectrum. The hydrophilic surfaces on which sunlight makes EZ water are more effective if they are colored (Pollack 2015). The important photosensitive porphyrins are pigmented. From the beginning, color has been an influence in the development of life. Ironically, it took billions of years for eyes to evolve that could see light and color.

ATMOSPHERE AND LIFE

Originally, living organisms had to rely on glycolysis or fermentation to obtain energy from glucose. This is a very slow and ineffective method for generating energy. In plants, a new method evolved to generate energy from sunlight and glucose. This relied on the chlorophyll molecule that, as noted above, breaks down carbon dioxide in the presence of water and sunlight to create glucose and oxygen as a by-product. This generates the oxygen in the atmosphere that animals breathe in and use to generate their energy. The oxygen in the atmosphere is attracted to the iron in the hemoglobin (another porphyrin) in animal blood, but the transfer itself is facilitated by yet another porphyrin-based enzyme, cytochrome oxidase. Animals expire carbon dioxide, which plants take in, creating a cycle that supports the biosphere in which all life flourishes.

Efficient Nature did not need to invent anything new: it uses the porphyrin ring to process oxygen in many different situations. The porphyrin ring includes chlorophyll, heme, and the cytochrome enzymes. Furthermore, Nature uses porphyrins to move electrons in bioelectricity. This family of molecules is as essential for life as oxygen, but is little appreciated. I did not understand the importance of porphyrins until I read a comment made by Arthur Firstenberg.

> Porphyrins are the very special molecules that interface between oxygen and life. They are responsible for the creation, maintenance, and recycling of all of the oxygen in our atmosphere: they make possible the release of oxygen from carbon dioxide by plants, the extraction of oxygen back out of the air by both plants and animals, and the use of that oxygen by living things to burn carbohydrates, fats, and proteins for energy. (Firstenberg 2016, 136)

Firstenberg also asks, How could we not know about these all-important molecules? Why are they not a household word like *chlorophyll* or *hemoglobin*? This is a good illustration of perspective, which was discussed in the introduction. It is easy to leave out the important facts—to not even know about them—but this will create holes in our perspective.

Clean air consists primarily of oxygen (about 70 percent), nitrogen (about 27 percent), water vapor, and a trace of carbon dioxide contributed by the breath of oxygen-breathing animals. Oxygen (O_2), whether in water or air, supplies a necessary component for fire or heat to exist, so it is crucial in both mineral and organic chemistry. Large amounts of fuel and oxygen, hit by a spark, produce fire, but the mere insertion of a few oxygen atoms into a substance causes a chemical breakdown and the release of energy—a controlled, smoldering fire. This is called *oxidation,* or in common speech, *weathering* if it is destructive and *metabolism* if it contributes to organic life.

The organism uses oxidation to break down and transform substances chemically; however, oxygen is constantly seeking to break down the organism itself, so parts are oxidizing (like the darkening of red meat), leading ultimately to the death of the living tissue. Oxidation releases energy until finally it brings about total release, or death. The removal of oxygen is called *reduction* and is used by the body to cut down on destructive oxidation. The metabolism, or ongoing hum of life in the organism, depends on constant oxidation and reduction, but eventually the former will triumph over the later. Oxygen has been called the sickle of the Lord of Death, but it is tamed and used by the living organism before the living being finally cannot resist the relentless push of oxidation and is devoured.

Oxygen is a highly active element that easily combines with or breaks into molecules to form new compounds with a release of energy in the form of heat. This process not only provides some of the chemical changes necessary to undertake digestion and metabolism but also the energy necessary to facilitate building (anabolism) as well as breaking down (catabolism). This includes the basic metabolism of the carbohydrates necessary for life undertaken by animals.

$$(6)\ O_2 + C_6H_{12}O_6 \text{ (glucose)} > \text{energy} + (6)\ H_2O + (6)\ CO_2$$

This reaction is facilitated by the enzyme cytochrome c, another porphyrin. Plant photosynthesis works in the opposite direction, as mentioned above.

$$\text{sunlight} + (6)\ H_2O + (6)\ CO_2 < C_6H_{12}O_6 + (6)\ O_2$$

We have observed the presence of carbon in all these chemical equations. It is like the substrate on which oxygen and hydrogen operate to make and remove energy. The principle carbon compounds used for this process are carbon dioxide, carbohydrates, sugars, and lipids (CH and CHO compounds). The carbon molecule is like a little "stick doll" or manikin that gets dressed up and undressed to store and release energy.

Although it does not appear in these reactions, nitrogen is essential for all of them to take place. Nitrogen is about as inert as oxygen is active, so it keeps the oxygen in the atmosphere from spontaneously exploding. Oxygen is too reactive by itself, so this hidden component of the air is just as necessary for life, even though it does not directly undertake any chemical operations in the atmosphere. However, it enters into the porphyrins and proteins that are so necessary for biological life to occur. Nitrogen is like the anvil the blacksmith beats on to form differently shaped instruments out of oxygen, hydrogen, carbon, and sometimes nitrogen itself. It is the basic element in protein, from which the body makes its "tools."

ORGANIC AND INORGANIC CHEMISTRY

These four chemical elements (O, H, C, N) constitute the building blocks of organic chemistry; they make up about 96.5 percent of the weight of the human body. Of this, 65 percent is oxygen, 18.5 percent is hydrogen, 9.5 percent is carbon, and 3.2 percent is nitrogen. The human body is 60 percent water. These four elements are called the *organic* elements because their presence and activities characterize organic life. The remaining 3.35 percent of elements found in the organism are called *inorganic* because they are active in both the mineral world and the organic world. Calcium constitutes about 1.5 percent of this, phosphorus 1 percent, and the rest altogether make up about 0.85 percent.

The most active of the inorganic elements in the living being are the electrolytes, which control the interaction of fluids and solids. The most common of these are dissociated H_2O, namely H+ and OH− ions. Others are calcium, sodium, magnesium, potassium (all positively charged), chloride, phosphorus, and sulfur (all negative). They will come up later in this chapter, in the discussion of the acidity and alkalinity of the matrix, but we will not follow them out in detail right now.

Oxygen (O)

This is the most abundant element in our environment. It is present in the atmosphere, water, earth, and all life-forms. Half the weight of the mineral world is oxygen, four-fifths of the vegetable, and more than half of the animal. More than half the atoms on Earth are oxygen.

Although it has no color, odor, or taste, oxygen is the most active of all the elements, easily combining with all of them except fluorine. It has nearly as hard a time with nitrogen, the great stabilizer or anvil of organic life. Because oxygen is so widely available and so reactive, compounds exposed to it in air or water are readily acted on and decomposed. This activity is known to us as weathering, rusting, decomposition, rotting, burning, or oxidation. If it happens slowly and the substance is fairly inert and hard for oxygen to get into, the substance slowly weathers or rusts. If a substance is more reactive, it rots or decomposes, but if it is highly reactive, it can be set on fire. If it is extraordinarily reactive, it can spontaneously burst into flame.

The fast progress of rust shows us how attractive iron is to oxygen, so (with the help of the porphyrin cytochrome oxidase) the iron in the porphyrin heme molecule pulls the oxygen out of the air into our lungs and binds it until the oxygen is brought to the capillary bed. The matrix is more attractive to oxygen than iron, so oxygen is pulled off the hemoglobin, through the porous capillary membranes into the milieu intérieur, and onward to the mitochondria in the cells, which use it to oxidize glucose to make energy.

Several basic health problems can be noted right here.

Free radicals are molecules that are unstable and therefore attract oxygen, which rips them apart. This results in out-of-bounds oxidation: the cells and tissues may be broken down, not just waste products. This results in inflammation of the tissue, with accompanying symptoms: heat, swelling, redness, and tenderness. Inflammation is the "mother of all disease." *Antioxidants* are molecules that stabilize the free radicals and cut down on systemic inflammation. One example is flavonoids, many of which come from fruit, which we do, in fact, on our macroscopic level, experience as cooling.

If not enough glucose is being consumed, the body breaks down lipids into glucose, and if not enough of them are available, it breaks down protein: that's when we start losing weight. All of this is facilitated by enzymes, including cytochrome c.

Another problem is more serious. Remember that the original forms of life, before the appearance of plants, were organisms that inefficiently generated energy from glycolysis—the fermentation of glucose? This was done without oxygen, because photosynthesis and hemoglobin did not yet exist. So it turns out that when oxygen is not present, cells revert to this primitive form of energy production and then begin to grow independently of the healthy cells, becoming cancer cells. They still depend on signals received from the GRS to know what to do, but they are using the system rather than being controlled by it.

Oxygen is the basis of the healthy transformation, feeding, and survival in the cell or organism. Yet, at the same time, oxygen is also constantly trying to insert itself into the chemical bonds of the living tissue itself. It "sticks its nose, as it were, into almost every other element's business," wrote the herbalist Edward Shook (1978, 67). Therefore, it is also the element that breaks down and kills the organism.

An example of the effect of oxygen can be seen on our own skin. Sun exposure causes oxidation, weathering, or what we call "aging" of the skin, resulting in rough, coarse, broken-up skin. Miners, who remain in the ground and away from sunlight, have smooth, ageless skin because they are not exposed to the sun.

Not only does oxygen cause inflammation by healthy and unhealthy oxidation, it also forms bonds with some elements that result in the production of the acid wastes of the body, particularly phosphate $(-OP_4)$, sulfate $(-OS_2)$, and carbonic acid (CO_2).

Oxygen, or the acid maker, has its name from its capacity for uniting with other substances. Of hydrogen it makes water; of nitrogen

various oxides and potent acids; of sulphur some of the most powerful acids; of carbon, phosphorus, arsenic, iron, and many other metals, active acids, each with its own properties. With most of these
an effect of union with oxygen is to produce the heat and light
which we associated with combustion. (Worcester 1889, 197)

Because it is so reactive, oxygen is needed by life-forms to help
them break down substances into compounds required for living. It also
breaks down waste products into less active, denatured "junk" that can
easily be moved out of the cell and organism via the waters of the body,
themselves made out of oxygen and hydrogen. Deep within the organism, the cells are able to control and harness the combustible oxygen,
using it to break down substances and generate energy. Thus, cells need
a constant flow of oxygen.

To provide this constant flow, oxygen is inhaled into the lungs,
going to the smallest units of the lungs, the alveoli, and is then attracted
across the pulmonary membrane to the hemoglobin in the blood's red
cells in the capillaries of the lungs. The hemoglobin releases CO_2 and
picks up the oxygen. The oxygenated blood is carried through the lungs,
to the left side of the heart, and on again to the arterial system and to
the capillaries, where CO_2 is so attracted to the hemoglobin that the
oxygen is released in favor of a "new lover." The CO_2 travels through
the veins back to the right side of the heart and to the lungs, from
which it is expelled into the atmosphere. Dumped off the hemoglobin,
the oxygen molecules move through the inner ocean of the body, the
interstitial fluids, until they come to a cell that needs them and draws
them inside it.

Nitrogen (N)

Nitrogen is classified as a noble gas because it does not easily form
bonds with other elements. It possesses eight electrons that fill the
eight basic orbital shells of the atom entirely, making little room for
electrons from other atoms to gain a foothold. However, it does form

an extremely stable compound with the hydrogen atom (one nucleus, one electron) called an *amine*—four hydrogen atoms attached to one nitrogen. This compound combines with other compounds to form *amino acids,* the basic building blocks of proteins. Amino acids are also very stable, allowing reliable chemistry to be carried on generation after generation so that even today we still possess some of the same basic protein chains as the original cells of life. One of these building blocks, ribonucleic acid (RNA), which is present in all living cells, also is stable and continually produces the same "basic commodities," including GAGs and PGs.

Because of its stability, nitrogen is found in vast quantities in the atmosphere, where it prevents the oxygen from blowing up the planet. Similarly, in organic life-forms, its stability is used to prevent oxidation and preserve the integrity of compounds. While hydrogen, oxygen, and carbon are found in unlimited supplies in the soil, nitrogen must be supplied by dead organic material, fertilizer, or compost.

> It seems to have no love for combining with oxygen, being mixed with it in the air for an indefinite time without union in any degree. By various organic processes it is combined with oxygen, hydrogen, carbon, and a little sulphur, of which elements all tissues and muscles in animal bodies are composed; also the grains and other nitrogenized kinds of food, by which such tissues are nourished. From the decomposition of such compounds, other compounds of nitrogen exist, as ammonia, nitrous and nitric acids, saltpeter, which is nitric acid and potash, and the numerous explosives which are made of nitric acid with carbon compounds. The power of these seems to arise from the quantity of oxygen lightly held by the nitrogen, and set free by heat or a blow to unite with other substances. (Worcester 1889, 198)

The porphyrin ring is also built on the diagram of a square, like the amino acid. The square or equal-sided cross, when it appears in chemistry, is the "signature" of nitrogen because its four orbital shells produce stable compounds that are four-sided or four-pronged. It is not surprising that nitrogen is found in the porphyrin rings that resist the siren call of oxidation and therefore are capable of controlling oxygen. The porphyrins include chlorophyll, heme, cytochrome c, cytochrome oxidase (which transfers oxygen from the air to the heme), cytochrome P450 (to facilitate hepatic oxidation), and myoglobin (facilitating oxygenation of the muscles).

Nitrogen is found throughout the body in the proteins that are built up out of the amino acids. They are the essential ingredient for reproduction and manufacture, and as such must be kept very stable. They also form structural material like the matrix polymers and fibers, out of which arise the entire connective tissue system, or structural system. There are two basic protein strands: deoxyribonucleic acid (DNA), the well-known basis for reproduction, from the single cell to the human being, and ribonucleic acid (RNA), which creates useful substances needed for survival in all organisms. Proteins bind with sugars to produce the glycosaminoglycans and proteoglycans of the matrix structure.

RNA proteins are like molds that produce—again and again—strands of protein that help direct life processes. DNA proteins are used to replicate the organism. If a protein becomes unstable and mutates, the signals and patterns will be changed and the organism will die or mutate. Because nitrogen is so stable, it is used to construct protein chains and help them maintain stability. It helps prevent cancer, a major cause of which is protein mutation. Nitrogen gives shape and integrity.

Connective tissue is composed of strands of protein, so that the bones, tendons, ligaments, cartilage, joints, and muscles are high in protein. When nitrogen levels are low and oxygen is not kept in check, these tissues are prone to inflammation. They are frequently the sites of autoimmune disease.

Nitrogen is colorless, odorless, and tasteless. Ironically, it helps pick up dark pigments from plants and makes people's complexion and hair dark, according to the alternative practitioner Victor G. Rocine (1856–1954). It is particularly found in the connective tissues, including the muscles, fibrous tissues, skin, and hair, and also in the blood. The loss of color in the hair and strength in the joints and bones indicates nitrogen loss. As soon as nitrogen leaves the body, tissues begin to decompose, and nitrogen is one of the first elements to go. And remember, it forms porphyrins that oppose the primitive energy-production habits of cancer cells by facilitating positive oxygenation.

Hydrogen (H)

Water is composed of hydrogen and oxygen. The blood vessels, lymphatics, synovial membranes, and nerve sheaths all contain specialized forms of water used by the body for different functions. The blood vessels carry water that is highly complexed with blood proteins, keeping it in the semipermeable vessels. This water is full of electrolytes, nutrients, red blood cells, white blood cells, platelets, and blood proteins. The viscosity is controlled by the potassium sulfate ion and prostaglandins. The watery portion of the blood is called the plasma. After the oxygen and nutrients and water for the cells have been dumped off in the capillaries, the venules absorb carbon dioxide (from cellular respiration of oxygen) and small waste products. However, large waste products, such as dead white blood cells and bacteria, pieces of cells and tissue, and so forth, are too large to be absorbed into the bloodstream and carried away. Hence, they are broken down by white blood cells and immune processes and then absorbed by the lymphatic capillaries. Eventually, the lymph is dumped into the bloodstream. Water is exuded into the epithelial cells of the mucosa and synovia to form mucin, digestive juices, synovia, and other functional fluids.

The CSF in the brain and nerve sheaths is an especially pure exudate of the blood, and it is separated off in the ventricles of the brain. It travels along the nerve sheaths and keeps them cool and lubricated. The nerve charge (electrons) jumps the nerve synapses through the CSF. A friend of mine who used to do spinal taps (before she became a chiropractor) says that CSF is a beautiful fluid that shines like starlight. It has its own beat (from the ventricles of the brain) and operates as an integrated fluid beating in syncopation from head to foot.

Medieval physicians thought that the soul resided in the ventricles of the brain, where the CSF is generated and collected. In a sense, they were right because the condition of the CSF strongly influences the psychic awareness of the individual. If the CSF is congested and bunched up, which often occurs due to whiplash and sometimes before the menses, withdrawal, introversion, and brooding can be caused. These conditions can also be induced due to psychic sensitivity. Severe bunching up of the CSF will cause chorea and spasms. A good remedy here is Black Cohosh (*Cimicifuga racemosa*).

Water is imbibed into the stomach and absorbed with food and other nutrients through the intestines. It is attracted into the body and all the way to the cell by sodium chloride. Some water is made in the interior from chemical reactions as well. Waste products are dumped from the cell into the interstitial fluids. According to alternative medicine (the cell salt theory), sodium sulphate disperses this water toward the outlets of the body. Sodium chloride in the water directs it through the kidneys and out of the body. Much also leaves through the skin and the colon. Water vapor and carbon dioxide leave through the lungs.

Carbon (C)

The cell needs fuel to burn. This is the sugar glucose, derived from the diet. It is usually derived from the digestion and metabolism of carbohydrates—or lipids or proteins if there is a shortage of carbohydrates. Inserting oxygen, the cell breaks apart the carbohydrate to produce heat or energy or fire. In addition, it also produces water and carbon dioxide as waste products that go back into the environment and into the great cycle of plant to animal to plant, or said another way, carbon dioxide to oxygen and back again.

Carbohydrates (CH) are water-soluble, but the cell also requires lipids, which are made of carbon, hydrogen, and oxygen (CHO) and are insoluble in water. Carbohydrates, lipids, and proteins together form the boundary membranes around the cells. There is a need for both water-soluble and oil-soluble surfaces and receptors in the cell membrane in order to keep a boundary with the outside world but also allow in foods with different solubilities.

The carbohydrates have several functions, but among others they function like glue to hold together the cell membrane in a flexible manner. Lipids, or fats and oils, are not water-soluble but are fat-soluble, so they enter into the construction of the boundary membrane that keeps the environmental water from coming into the cell and keeps the internal water remaining within the cell. Lipophilic receptors are also needed on the cell membrane, and proteins are needed as building materials to strengthen membranes and for recognition purposes.

Carbon is the "dust of the earth," a common, pedestrian substance, yet it is indispensable for the formation of organic substances. All sorts of compounds crucial for life processes are made from carbon. It can be combined to make many wonderful things, and it enters into two of the three basic foods of living organisms: carbohydrates (carbon and hydrogen) and lipids (carbon, hydrogen, and oxygen). When it is tweaked with various exotic elements and compounds, it forms organic molecules that have specific functions.

Carbon is tasteless and odorless. At room temperature, pure carbon is found in substances as diverse as diamonds and pencil lead. Here, pressure has made the difference. Heat, sunlight, and pressure act on it. Carbon is a highly passive substance, acted on by outside influences, rather than seeking out and causing change in other elements. Yet it is also fairly stable: water and air do not act on it, nor do alkalies and acids. As a building block, it forms compounds with other carbons or with hydrogen that are invaluable to life. The compounds thus formed become the basis for tweaking with more complex substances.

Carbon combines with other elements to form common substances in the earth such as limestone, dolomite, chalk, and coal. It will be noticed that all of these substances are derived from deposits of organic materials—shells, bones, leaves, and wood. Over half the plant world consists of carbon. It is left in these huge deposits by dead organisms that have collected it as a monument to its organic utility.

There are two basic pathways by which carbon enters the organic world. First, by the combination of carbon atoms with other carbon atoms, and second, by the combination of carbon with hydrogen. It is important in generating energy as well. Whenever carbon and oxygen are found together, heat is generated. In combination with hydrogen, it forms the carbohydrates, and with hydrogen and oxygen, it forms lipids. These two substances, with protein, are the basis of animal nutrition. Muscles contain large amounts of carbon.

When carbon is oxidized, it enters organic life-forms, where it is used, stored, or formed into essential molecules of life. Carbon dioxide is formed as a waste product of animal respiration.

Carbon and hydrogen together form carbohydrates, which are water-soluble. These are subdivided into two groups: the sugars and the starches. They are all characteristically sweet, except for the long chain sugars and starches, which taste bland (like mucus and wood). A variety of short-term sugars such as fructose (fruit sugar), glucose (grape sugar), lactose (milk sugar), and sucrose (refined cane sugar) are consumed as food, but all are broken down in the gastrointestinal tract into glucose and absorbed into the bloodstream, sent to the liver, and processed into glycogen, which is either stored in the liver for future use or sent to the muscles for storage and eventual use. Glycogen is changed back into glucose and used in massive doses by the cells for food to generate energy, which is measured in calories. The brain requires a huge, constant supply of blood. If this fails to arrive, there would be collapse and death; however, in such cases, adrenaline kicks in and stored glycogen is brought out of storage for use. That is why we feel an adrenaline rush when temporarily short on food. Too much sugar, on the other hand, causes high blood sugar levels and can cause a temporary overactivity of brain and muscles. The high blood sugar levels raise insulin levels until the sugar is absorbed. This can cause hyperinsulinemia and type 2 diabetes.

Starches are also broken down and made into glucose for use in the body. There are two kinds of starches: refined and unrefined. The former are quickly digested and quickly produce energy. Like sugar, refined starches produce a sudden, high blood sugar spike with the same deleterious effects. Unrefined starches, on the other hand, are difficult to digest, slow down the assimilation of glucose, require calories to be consumed, and lower the blood sugar spike. They also provide potassium, which is required for insulin to get glucose into the cell: one potassium, one sugar molecule. Thus, low potassium levels also cause high blood sugar levels.

When carbohydrates are eaten in too-large amounts, they are bound up with a glycerol molecule to become triglycerides. These are stored as fats in low-density lipoprotein (LDL) cholesterols, which are deposited in fat tissue or on arteries. Alternative nutritionists believe that the most damaging LDL cholesterol buildup in arteries is due to the overconsumption of carbohydrates, rather than fats and oils; the latter are blamed by conventional nutritionists.

Lipids, or fats and oils, consist of carbon and hydrogen, but they have some oxygen in a hydroxyl group (OH−) that causes them to become oil-soluble rather than water-soluble. Lipids are taken up in the food supply and assimilated into the lymphatic system and then the blood. According to alternative nutritionists, most of them are used for replacement parts by cells and tissues needing lipids. Some fatty acids are required for liver function. Conventional nutritionists blame them for arterial disease.

Long chain sugars (polysaccharides) in food are essentially the same as the polymers of the matrix inside the body. They are intentionally used as mucilages by herbalists to coat and sooth the mucosa of the gastrointestinal tract. They can enter into and replenish the "mortar" between the cells lining the tract, which is made by matrix polymers, and some of them can enter into the matrix through these membranes. Others are broken down for food; they are a hard-to-digest sugar that does not cause high blood sugar levels. An example of a food with mucilage in it is Okra.

Long chain starches form cellulose, a structural material used in plants to form wood. This is indigestible for human beings, though cows and other ruminants can digest grass that contains cellulose. Cellulose from plants passes through the human digestive system and is used as roughage to stimulate peristalsis in the intestines. It was once thought that cellulose and roughage were unnecessary. This is what sent V. E. Irons to prison for six months in 1956: claiming that roughage was necessary for healthy bowel movements. Later, this was proved to be true, and "whole grain" bread with unrefined carbohydrates was accepted as an important source of cellulose.

Electrolytes

The role of the electrolytes in controlling fluids, substances, and functions is widely recognized in modern medical science. Tests for the measurement of levels of electrolytes and fluids have long been used as basic diagnostic parameters. This knowledge fits hand in glove with our increasing understanding of the matrix and also with old-time medicine, which emphasized the regulation of the channels of fluid elimination. Due to the complexity of the subject, we will not be discussing electrolytes in depth in this book.

Electrolytes consist of two ions, one positively charged (having an extra electron) and one with a negative charge (seeking an electron). The positive ions are known as cations, the negative as anions. The electrolyte therefore has a neutral charge. This makes it stable in a solid form, but an electrolyte will dissolve in water to form a solution that is electrically conductive. The dissolved or dissociated ions are called *solutes*. The cations are drawn to the positive electrode, and the anions to the negative one, so the electrons travel from positive to negative, and this creates an electrical current. As mentioned, the major cations are hydrogen, sodium, potassium, and calcium; the common anions are phosphate, sulfate, chloride, and bicarbonate. Phosphorus and sulfur combine with oxygen to form the anions $-OP_4$ and $-OS_2$. The carbonic acid $(-HCO_2)$ produced as a waste from energy production in the cell recombines to form bicarbonate $(-HCO_3)$. The most common electrolytes are, therefore, sodium chloride (NaCl), sodium sulphate $(NaSO_2)$, sodium bicarbonate $(NaHCO_3)$, calcium phosphate $(CaOP_4)$, potassium sulfate (KSO_2), and magnesium ions.

ACID AND ALKALINE

As an environment, one of the most important factors in maintaining the homeostasis of the matrix is the balance of acidity and alkalinity, or pH levels. For perspective on this subject, I consulted a paper by Yoshinori Marunaka, who notes that pH levels in the matrix regulate various enzymes and the binding affinities of proteins, hormones, and neurotransmitters to their receptor sites. He says, "This means that pH of interstitial fluids plays one of the most important key roles in regulation of cell function" and the maintenance of homeostatic balance. But he adds that "unfortunately little information on pH of interstitial fluids is available" because it is hard to measure pH levels in the matrix and blood pH levels cannot be applied to the interstitial fluids (Marunaka 2015). So we don't have a lot of information on the pH level of the matrix, even though it is one of the most important factors in the maintenance of homeostasis inside the ECM.

The dissociation of water into hydrogen ions and hydroxyls sets up the basic acidity and alkalinity possible in the fluids of the living organism. This is modified by other ions. A predominance of H+ ions makes the solution alkaline; the hydroxyls make it acidic. The number of hydrogen ions present is measured on the pH scale: 7 is neutral, above 7 is alkaline or base (positive charge; high H+ ions), and below 7 is acidic (negative; low H+ ions). The limits of the scale are 0 and 14.

To give a sensory idea of pH levels, think of the following: a pH of 0 = battery acid, 1 = hydrochloric acid from the stomach,

2 = lemon juice, 3 = grapefruit juice, 4 = tomato juice and acid rain, 5 = black coffee, 6 = healthy urine and saliva, 7 = pure water, 8 = seawater, 8.4 = eggs, 9 = baking soda, and 14 = liquid drain cleaner.

A lot is made of the pH level of the body fluids in both conventional and alternative medicine, and rightly so, since the pH level reflects excesses and deficiencies of basic ingredients necessary for life, as well as setting up the environment in which they are processed. However, there is not agreement between professional and popular medicine about how to interpret, measure, or treat pH imbalances.

It is often stated in popular medicine that the "blood" is too acid or alkaline. The blood is actually heavily buffered and only fluctuates in the narrow band between 7.35 and 7.45 pH, so this is untrue. However, the term "blood" has long been used in folk medicine to mean "body fluids" in a general sort of way. It was used in this way for thousands of years in folk medicine before science came along, so we cannot really criticize people for speaking in this manner. However, it has to be understood that this is not a basis for scientific definition and communication.

Since the blood plasma becomes the interstitial fluid of the ECM and that becomes the lymph in the lymphatics, one would think that the acid/alkaline balance in the matrix would be fairly constant at the same level of the blood. However, it is not: the normal interstitial fluid pH level fluctuates between 6.60 and 7.60. The blood is heavily buffered and monitored by the kidneys, but the interstitial fluids need to vary in order to undertake the numerous physiological functions that occur within the matrix. If they were buffered, many metabolic processes could not occur. Lymph, although an eliminative fluid coming off the matrix, returns to the same basic pH level of the blood. Eliminative substances such as urine and saliva also fluctuate in pH, so they do not reflect the pH of the blood or lymph.

Under healthy conditions, cells generate hydrogen ions that, when extruded into the matrix, keep the pH level of interstitial fluids from becoming too acidic from other cellular waste in the form of carbonic acid, phosphates, and sulfates. The H+ ions are largely produced in the

Krebs cycle in the mitochondria of the cells. They bind with the carbonic acid to form bicarbonate, one of the important buffers of pH in the organism. From the matrix, H+ ions also diffuse into the blood, where they bind with protein buffers that act to maintain pH levels. The Ca++ ions in the bone act as a backup buffer system, going into a solution to pick up excess phosphate ions, which are either then reabsorbed back into the bone or deposited out pathologically as calcification in soft tissues. This helps to explain why medicinal plants like Boneset (*Eupatorium perfoliatum*) and Gravel Root (*Eupatorium,* now *Eutrochium purpureum*) have effects on bone repair, aberrant calcium deposition, and the movement of fluids and solutes across membranes.

The interstitial fluids and matrix polymers generally possess a slightly negative charge. This attracts sodium ions into the polymers, which are therefore coated with sodium. This in turn attracts the water molecules that keep the polymers hydrated. The polymers therefore act something like a sodium bank, the way the bones act for calcium.

Since water follows sodium—throw salt on the table on a humid day and collect the damp salt later—this ion is important in maintaining water levels in the matrix. Too much increases water retention and blood pressure. When a lower pH level in the matrix occurs, the sodium will be involved in buffering the fluids rather than attracting water into the polymers. Then, the polymers will become dehydrated and collapse in upon themselves, so there will be a combination of dry tissues and thin fluids. This may be the origin of the "high-walled pulse" of Ayurvedic medicine, where the vessel under the finger feels like a PVC tube and the blood inside it feels like a thin, watery fluid running through the pipe. For this condition, I give a salty mucilage like Marshmallow Root (*Althea officinalis*) or the homeopathic cell salt Natrum muriaticum (sodium chloride), usually in the 30C potency.

Understanding pH Fluctuation

When the digestive tract demands an acid to break down food, hydrogen ions and chloride ions are pulled out of the blood to produce hydrochloric acid (HCl). This creates an imbalance in the ECFs called the *alkaline tide* because of the loss of the Cl anion in large numbers. This is largely buffered by sodium bicarbonate, sodium phosphate, and the protein buffering system. Since less than 1 percent to 2 percent of the potassium (K) and calcium (Ca) are ever in solution in the ECFs and magnesium is only present in a trace amount, sodium (Na) is the main alkaline cation available for these buffer systems. However, from their depositories (potassium in the cells and calcium in the bones), these ions also influence the pH, but less so than sodium. A potassium deficiency pulls sodium into the cells, making it less available, while bone stores phosphates as calcium phosphate, contributing to the regulation of phosphate levels.

If interstitial fluids had pH-buffering proteins like albumin in the blood, the osmotic pressure of the interstitial fluids would increase, suppressing the passage of nutrients and metabolites from the blood across the capillary bed into the matrix. This is what happens when there are high sodium or calcium levels in the matrix. This is where calcium channel blockers are used to keep down the calcium and sodium levels in the matrix—and the blood pressure.

Marunaka found that lowered pH levels in the interstitial fluids often accompanied insulin resistance, the precursor to type 2 diabetes. On the endocrine level, the predominance of mineralocorticoids in the adrenal cortex keeps up the sodium level and the alkalinity, while the glucocorticoid cortisol suppresses the sodium level and increases the glucose level and acidity in the blood.

An acid/alkaline imbalance may not originate in the matrix, but in the mitochondria. Patients with type 2 diabetes are believed to have lower mitochondrial function. Thus, they will not make as much of the H+ that maintains the pH level of the ECFs. Marunaka explains, "Although our studies have not yet clarified the molecular mechanism causing lowered pH of interstitial fluids, these phenomena would be due to dysfunction or hypo-function of mitochondria in diabetes mellitus" (Marunaka 2015). Low production of energy in the mitochondria affects the charge on the cell membrane, which in turn changes the receptivity to various GRS signals. This is where the cell danger response theory comes into play: when the cell is under attack, as in inflammation, the mitochondria shift from production of energy to cell membrane protection. In this instance, the cell is acting back toward the matrix rather than operating wholly under matrix control.

Insulin resistance usually results from insufficient uptake of glucose into skeletal muscle, causing a prolonged high blood glucose level. Since insulin-like growth factor 1 (IGF-1) is the major type of insulin used to send glucose to skeletal muscles and is also identical to the *sulfation factor* that adds the sulfate to the glycosaminoglycans, the condition of the matrix and type 2 diabetes are going to be very intimately intertwined. Marunaka does not mention this, but it is generally believed in conventional medicine that an increased level of alkaline salts increases the level of IGF-1, which would bring down the blood sugar level and maintain a healthy matrix and connective tissue system.

One thing that Marunaka found that is interesting is that the pH level of the interstitial fluid around the hippocampus may be lower in people with type 2 diabetes, suggesting diminished neuronal activity of the brain. This in turn may result in dementia and Alzheimer's disease. Other factors related to type 2 diabetes also occur in people with this condition, but Marunaka suggests the "maintenance of the interstitial fluid pH at the normal level," or a return to that level, "would be a key factor" in developing treatment for these conditions (Marunaka 2015).

Holistic Treatments for pH Dysregulation

Biomedicine keeps close tabs on the pH level of the blood, while popular medicine tends to prefer the much easier measurement of pH in the saliva and urine. This can be done at home with litmus paper, rather than at a lab drawing blood. Neither, however, accurately measures the condition in the matrix.

How are we to treat acidosis or alkalosis?

Both biomedicine and complementary and alternative medicine

oppose the long-term use of alkaline antacids to reduce irritating stomach acidity because these agents cause the body to secrete more and more hydrochloric acid to digest them—leading to greater acid secretion in the stomach. This suggests an explanation for why acidic fruits are used in alternative medicine for treating chronic internal acidosis. Not only do they contain healthy amounts of the alkaline salts found in living tissue, but they also reduce the secretion of hydrochloric acid by the stomach and the resulting alkaline tide that occurs internally from the loss of the chlorine into the stomach. So, ironically, acidic foods would tend to moderate pH levels in people with high stomach acidity. An example of this type of therapy is the consumption of vinegar or honey and vinegar on a regular basis as advocated by the Vermont country doctor D. C. Jarvis in his 1959 book *Folk Medicine*. Another such approach would be the consumption of umeboshi plums in Japanese cuisine.

Nineteenth-century doctors generally associated an acidic condition of the stomach with a red or dark red tongue, while an alkaline condition was associated with a pale tongue. This is pretty easy to understand since a red tongue will be associated with the kind of irritation we would see with a high stomach acid level, while the pale tongue and oral cavity would fit with very poor secretion. The condition of the internal body fluids would be opposite that of the stomach, since the withdrawal of chlorine from the interior creates an alkaline tide in the ECFs. When acidic secretion in the stomach is low, the tongue is pale and the internal fluids are more acidic. The standard treatments for these conditions were acids (red tongue) and alkalies (pale tongue) (Scudder 1874).

"ONE HALF THE FLASH OF LIGHTNING"

The importance of electron transport in GRS signaling, piezoelectricity, and nerve transmission has already been noted. Despite the all-pervading presence of electromagnetic phenomena in life processes, they are almost completely overlooked as a topic in pathology and therapy.

Over the last seventy-five years, the subject has been largely consigned to oblivion. However, electricity is everywhere present within living organisms and must be considered as another primal overarching component of life. It is like the fifth element to the four elements of water, fire, air, and earth.

It was not originally my intention to include electricity in my account of the ECM, but I was converted from this myopic view by Arthur Firstenberg's unique, invaluable, and highly readable book, *The Invisible Rainbow: The History of Electricity and Life* (2016). Electricity—that is, the flow of electrons along a conductive surface (a semiconductor)—is crucial to life on every level, from the cellular to the neurological. The polymers of the matrix and the cytoskeleton of the cell maintain electrical potential charges that change when the conditions of life change. The movement of connective tissue creates "static electricity" or piezoelectricity that travels along fascia, tendons, bones, and other structures of the body. This is the basis of the biomechanical regulatory system. When we think of bioelectricity, however, it is usually in the form of our nervous system. Actually, the movement or exchange of every electron in the body, the basis of all biochemical activity, is electrical.

When we think of electricity in the environment, it is mostly in the form of lightning, so it is no wonder if it is difficult for us to imagine or value the insensible transfer of electrons in the matrix or along the bones, in plants, or through the ground. As if to remind us, from time to time that our body is electrical, we get a shock from static electricity. The fifth element is a trickster.

Electricity has only been a subject of study since 1746, when some "wild static electricity" was "captured" in a Leyden jar in the Netherlands. When it was first observed—with its literally shocking effect—it was thought possible that this was the "vital force" that many natural philosophers had been arguing for or against. It has been dismissed as such since electricity is found in so many different settings, organic and inorganic, or for other reasons, but it does have an extremely close relationship to life processes. It is always present when there is movement or animation of living things, from the exchange of electrons to changes in charge levels to the trickle of electrons along bones to normal neuromuscular movement to the shock of static electricity or lightning.

Once we understand that electricity is fundamental to biological function and that all changes in health and disease will be accompanied by changes in electrical charges and movements, we begin to appreciate how important this field is to the maintenance of public and individual health. Yet, it is almost entirely ignored.

> By ignoring the fact that most biological functions are electrically controlled the medical profession remains ignorant to the fact that the low frequency electromagnetic fields, generated by most of the electronic or electrical gadgetry of our day, will superimpose over these natural bioelectric fields, thereby altering their functions. (Barefoot and Reich 2002, 5)

I have a difficult time remembering basic chemistry, so pardon my return to middle school science class. Matter is composed of tiny positive and negative charges—the protons and electrons. They are attracted to each other and each has an equal charge, so protons and electrons combine to form atoms. The simplest atom is hydrogen, with one of each; more protons and electrons produce larger atoms, some of which have unequal charges since they lack the electrons necessary to balance the protons. To remedy this, these elements are attracted to other elements to form more stable, balanced compounds or molecules. Groups of molecules together form the substances we see in the world. Because protons and electrons seek balance for stability, these large bodies are electrically neutral, so that the world we live in is normally electrically balanced. However, within many substances, including organic and inorganic bodies, electrons move from place to place. Whether fast or slow, this constitutes electricity. Also, differences in charge can build up; a bunch of electrons can pile up in one area. Their discharge constitutes visible or sensible electricity. A difference of charge between positive and negative poles is called *magnetism,* not referring to an iron magnet, per se, but to the general property of attraction between the poles.

Porphyrins, Electricity, and Life

In the spring of 2019, I went to visit Arthur Firstenberg, one of the most interesting voices in alternative medicine. I call his concepts "alternative" and not "complementary" because, if ever there was a department of medicine that was ignored, it is the influence of electricity on biological organisms. Even herbs are generally conceded to have some medicinal power, but electricity—despite its sometimes awesome show of force—has been strangely dismissed.

If we are going to discuss electricity, we need to discuss porphyrins because these substances not only generate and control oxygen but also facilitate the movement of electrons in the body. I did not understand the importance of porphyrins until I read Arthur's book, *The Invisible Rainbow* (2017). Despite their ubiquity and significance in biology, porphyrins are hardly mentioned in popular or professional scientific medicine.

Porphyrins are strangely symmetrical, squarish but circular molecules and are found in both inorganic and organic forms. They are photosensitive, a property associated with pigmentation, so that the molecules they enter are often colorful, such as chlorophyll and hemoglobin. Porphyrins are also the essential component in myoglobin, the protein that delivers oxygen from the bloodstream to the muscle cells and the source of the pink-red color of muscle.

Porphyrins are also important constituents of several extremely significant enzymes. Cytochrome c helps with the oxidation of carbohydrates, lipids, and proteins, to facilitate their digestion, metabolism, and elimination. Cytochrome oxidase, as the name indicates, facilitates the uptake of oxygen in the lungs. Cytochrome P450 is the enzyme that is essential for the detoxification of lipids in the liver (and all cells), including many environmental toxins. And finally, there is the heme component of hemoglobin and the porphyrin component in myoglobin.

Since porphyrins catalyze the movement of electrons along all tissues, they facilitate the electric charge in the matrix, on the cell membranes, and inside the cells, also the piezoelectric charge on the bones and connective tissue, and finally the nerves. When a break occurs—an incursion into the matrix, bone fracture, nerve injury—the flow of electrons facilitated by porphyrins is temporarily halted. Usually, it starts up quickly, but if it does not we have wounds that do not heal "by the first intention," to use the archaic phrase. The break remains open, unconjoined. Modern research—and now orthopedic therapy—have shown that running a mild electric current along bones can cure the nonunion of a fracture and also improve healing of trauma to the nervous system. Changes in electrical charges on the matrix result from acupuncture stimulation, so it appears that a "broken circuit" in the matrix, due to suspended activity of the porphyrins, would constitute a type of pathology that acupuncture acts on when it is not also acting on the biomechanical regulatory system or the nervous system. The technology used by orthopedists to facilitate electron flow has in fact been used by acupuncturists.

Static energy caused by movements over and against various types of connective tissue generates the low charge of piezoelectricity that travels along the bones. Calcium and carbon slow down whatever conductivity the phosphorus in the bone has, so bones are very poor semiconductors. However, it turns out that bones have trace amounts of metallic molecules that enhance this capacity, so that these slow electric currents can move along the skeletal system.

The remedy of choice for a "break in the circuit" in the piezoelectric current is St. John's Wort (*Hypericum perforatum*). I had a client who had a fracture in a bone in the wrist that wasn't healing after six weeks in a cast, but three remedies started the healing of the fracture within two or three days. Mullein is a specific for problems in the complex little bones of the wrist, ankles, and spine, Boneset is for setting bones, and St. John's Wort for reestablishing piezoelectric flow.

St. John's Wort contains pigmented compounds that are in fact proto-porphyrins and acts on almost every function in the body that involves porphyrins. Famously, *Hypericum* cannot be used with many drugs because it fires up the cytochrome P450 pathway, causing the metabolism of drugs too rapidly in the liver.

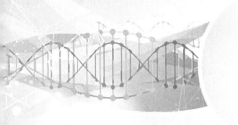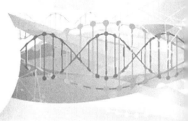

3

The Ground Substance
Architecture of the Matrix

Physiologists . . . must take account of the harmony of this whole, even while trying to get inside, so as to understand the mechanism of its every part.

CLAUDE BERNARD (1980, 89)

Now that we know the "background" of the matrix, let's move to the foreground—the polymers, fibers, and structures that occupy the matrix. An easy-to-read review article on the components of the ECM that I have relied on is "The Extracellular Matrix at a Glance," by Christian Frantz, Kathleen M. Stewart, and Valerie M. Weaver (2010).

GLYCOSAMINOGLYCANS

The ground substance, to review, is composed largely of glycosaminoglycans (GAGs: amino acids and sugars) bound to protein spines to form proteoglycans (PGs: protein sugars) that unfold into feather-like or wing-like structures when hydrated, then fold back together again when dried out. The PG structures are the major units of the matrix and are called matrisomes.

Each GAG is a polymer, that is to say, a long, unbranching chain of molecules only one molecule wide. They attract water, so the naked eye sees nothing more than a hydrated gel. In animals, this gel is interlaced with connective tissue fibers that add strength, flexibility, structure, and mobility. Other types of fibers occur in plants, combining with PGs to form the mucilage so familiar to the herbalist. The three major components of the matrix are, therefore, the GAGs, the PGs, and connective tissue fibers.

The basic unit of a GAG is an amino acid sugar (either glucosamine or galactosamine) that combines with an uronic acid sugar. There are some variations. Keratan sulfate has a different kind of amino acid, and dermatan sulfate has a variation in the uronic acid end. The unification of the amino acid sugar and the uronic acid sugars produces what is called a *disaccharide unit.*

Long chains of disaccharides are combined to form *polysaccharides* (meaning "many sugars"). This is a term many herbalists are familiar with as a major constituent of plant life. Disaccharides compose the polysaccharides made by enzymes in the cells, so no two GAGs are identical in size and all are polymers. Because of their physical properties, GAGs were originally known as *mucopolysaccharides,* a term that is still in use in herbal medicine. The mixture of GAGs and matrix fibers constitutes what we call *mucilage* in herbal medicine. Herbalists are among the few professionals who use mixed, natural selections of GAGs in their work.

The disaccharides, with some variations, are attached to a sulfate, except for hyaluronic acid (HA), the most primitive and original of all GAGs. HA is made by enzymes in the plasma membrane of the cell. Later on, cells developed an apparatus to make GAGs. Long before anybody knew what it did, scientists named this structure the Golgi body (later known as the Golgi apparatus). It manufactures the sulfated GAGs, sending them forth in little bubbles (vacuoles) to the surface of the cell for release into the matrix or keeping them inside for use in the structural material of the cell. The major sulfated GAGs are chondroitin sulfate, dermatan sulfate, keratan sulfate, and heparan sulfate/heparin.

GAGs have a highly negative charge, which gives them a capacity for bonding with other compounds. They are highly attractive to water and sodium, both of which coat the polymers. The attractiveness to water is enhanced by the addition of the sulfate, a process called *sulfation*. Chondroitin sulfate is the most common GAG in the body and enters into the composition of cartilage. Dermatan sulfate has a different uronic acid component and was formerly called chondroitin sulfate B. It is also found in connective tissue, especially in the skin, tendons, heart valves, vessel linings, lungs, and intestinal mucosa. Keratan sulfate contains a slightly different GAG. Physiologists originally found it only in the cornea, but it has also now been found elsewhere in structural tissue. Heparan sulfate contains distinct sulfated and nonsulfated regions. It is similar in structure to heparin, a substance with a wide variety of actions that is best known for its blood-thinning capacities. Both are made by the same enzymes, depending on the signals received, and there are intermediate types, so they are now classified as a single substance. They are involved in the immune function of the matrix. Heparin possesses the highest negative charge of any known biological molecule, so it contributes significantly to the negative electrical potential charge on the matrix polymers.

Sulfation Factor (IGF-1)

Sulfation factor, a remarkable and extremely important element of the matrix, is not usually mentioned in textbooks on the subject—not even by Pischinger. I owe my knowledge of it to Dr. William B. Ferril, a holistic medical doctor and author of *The Body Heals* (2004). Sulfation factor is now an old-fashioned and forgotten name. It was renamed "insulin-like growth factor 1" (IGF-1) when more of its properties were discovered. However, this caused the connection with sulfation to be forgotten.

Sulfation factor instructs the disaccharide to combine with a sulfate. This makes the resulting GAG "slippery" or "slimy," reminding us that GAGs are the major ingredients in mucin or mucus and mucilage. GAGs lubricate linings and cover them with a protective film. For example, the hydrochloride acid in the stomach can't eat through the gastric wall because it is covered with an adhesive, thick film of GAGs.

Sulfation factor consists of seventy amino acids bound in a chain and bridged in three places by disulfides. It is similar to insulin in structure and performs a similar function, making possible the pickup of glucose by the muscles, the same way insulin makes sugar available to nonmuscular tissue. It is also a growth factor that is very important in childhood, spurts in production during puberty, levels off to maintain tissues in adulthood, and declines in old age. Production is stimulated by human growth hormone, and IGF-1 is itself a hormone produced by the liver, as well as in local areas. In people with cancer, IGF-1 levels are high, promoting cancer cell growth and the pickup of glucose by the cancer cells.

Ferril points out that changing the name from sulfation factor to IGF-1 "created a disconnect in medical understanding" (2004, 161). The former name emphasized the manufacture of the all-important GAG polymers that form the substratum of the matrix, while the latter associated the substance with the equally large arena of sugar metabolism. Ferril points out the new name had adverse associations. Since cancers feed off glucose, it "helps instill fear of the same molecule being a growth factor for cancer cells." As a result, "many physicians remain unaware" of the important sulfation application "because the vocabulary uniting this association has been" lost.

I fully agree. I didn't find anything about IGF-1 and the matrix in regular medical literature until Ferril's careful analysis pierced the veil for me. One can find this sort of change in nomenclature completely obscuring or altering thinking in many fields. Once again, the importance of perspective comes to the fore.

In healthy people, IGF-1 is found in a 100:1 ratio with regular insulin, and if it is low, the latter must rise in compensation. It helps sugar enter the muscles so the active person uses more of it than the inactive. IGF-1 works in tandem with potassium, just like regular insulin. For every molecule of sugar and insulin, a potassium ion is needed to get the sugar in the cell. Consequently, potassium deficiency raises blood sugar levels. In addition, it has a negative effect on IGF-1 levels and is associated with muscular weakness and, eventually, atrophy.

IGF-1 is created in the liver under the influence of human growth hormone. This hormone is allied with the mineralocorticoid side of adrenal cortex functions (Selye 1956). It is therefore associated with people of the more buff constitutional type that results from the heat generation and pro-inflammatory orientation of the mineralocorticoids. These hormones are opposed by the anti-inflammatory glucocorticoid hormones of the adrenal cortex. This is why sulfation factor is associated with exercise, muscles, and the more buff *pitta* constitution. This constitution is high in calcium, potassium, and magnesium, which are all needed when there is much muscular activity. Sulfur is common in all foods, so it is not usually thought of as a limiting factor.

A low IGF-1 level probably causes the classic diabetic constitution, which results in a person with a thick apple-shaped torso, smaller limbs and hands and feet, smaller muscles, muscular weakness, and a propensity to type 2 diabetes. This constitution occurs because there is less IGF-1 going to the muscles of the limbs, resulting in diminished growth of the arms and legs, but more regular insulin, which activates the visceral organs of digestion and metabolism in the torso. A high level of sulfation factor with lower levels of regular insulin creates strong arms and legs, so these people should be tall, strong, large-handed, boney, muscular, and sinewy. Among the male representatives, I would think of Max von Sydow, John Wayne, and most basketball players; among the females, we would look for the tall figure so desirable in the "fashion model type," such as Nancy Kerrigan, Cindy Crawford, and Julia Roberts. Women with this type also have large hands. One can see the results of the higher calcium levels in these people. Victor G. Rocine, who based constitutional assessment on the essential elements, would have called these calcium-bearing constitutions the thick and the tall.

Because of the disconnect in medical science, we don't find much in the literature about what sulfation factor does. I had to go back to the cell salt model of alternative medicine to gain more insight. When Dr. Wilhelm Schüessler came up with the cell salt theory, which is now a sort of subdivision of homeopathy; one of his twelve salts was sodium sulfate ($NaSO_4$), also called Natrum sulphuricum. In a gross material form, this compound is known as Glauber's salts and is highly laxative, making the bowel walls slippery and lubricated. This is explained by its action on GAGs, making them more abundant and slippery so that the mucosal linings (intestines, gallbladder ducts, respiratory tract, etc.) are lubricated and nourished. It should also act on the GAGs in the ECM, making them more flexible and hydrated, thus increasing elimination from the matrix. Sodium sulfate therefore has a reputation in the cell salt system for cleansing the inner waters around the cells. Sodium sulfate and potassium sulfate both seem to make the solutes move more readily in the fluids.

Hyaluronic Acid

The most important of all GAGs is the original and most primitive: hyaluronic acid. No two hyaluronins are identical in size or structure since they are made by enzymes in the cell membrane rather than from templates. They are secreted into the matrix by the enzyme, until, at some point, the chain breaks off. These molecules are huge and have a high binding capacity, making them highly attractive to water and capable of ion exchange with it. They require a huge amount of water to completely hydrate and unfold.

The negative electric potential they carry gives hyaluronins a high capacity for bonding with proteins. They are bound by protein linker molecules to proteins to create large, fanlike proteoglycans that are primary structural units in the matrix. This allows for the development of different topographies (shapes and sizes) in the matrix, and therefore constitutes the evolutionary starting point for the distinctive tissues and organs that developed in the higher multicellular organisms (Pischinger 1991).

Hyaluronins possess the ability to regulate cell division and movement and to inhibit excessive or premature division, so that they have the strongest regulatory effect of any of the matrix GAGs on developing organs and tissues and also inhibit the development and spread of cancer.

As far back as 1966, it had been observed that the resistance to the spread of a malignant tumor would be increased in the presence of a strong ground substance, HA in particular. In that year, a Scottish surgeon, Ewan Cameron, published a book, *Hyaluronidase and Cancer*. Some bacteria, and probably all malignant neoplasms, produce an enzyme called hyaluronidase that breaks down this GAG so that the tumor can spread. To visualize the action of this enzyme, think of rattlesnake venom. It too possesses hyaluronidase and breaks down the ground substance in order for the venom to spread. In addition, some and perhaps all neoplasms, release another enzyme, collagenase, which breaks down collagen fibrils that are partly built up from the sulfated GAGs such as chondroitin, elastin, and dermatan. This phenomenon led to the introduction of glucosamine sulfate and chondroitin sulfate in the 1990s in order to strengthen the matrix against the spread of cancer. A "side effect" of this treatment was the widespread improvement in arthritic conditions, which will be mentioned below.

Although all of the matrix polymers are important, none has the sphere of action of HA. Pischinger notes:

> Compared to other biopolymers, hyaluronic acid in aqueous solution covers a very large domain. . . .
>
> This "domain" has a significant role in determining the "molecular sieve character," as well as the viscoelastic, shock-absorbing and

energy absorbing behavior of the extracellular matrix. (Pischinger 1991, 46, 52)

The ground substance created in this way possesses a simple defensive mechanism: it acts as a sieve to mechanically prevent the passage of large molecules into the matrix. The outward pressure (isomosis) exerted by the viscoelastic power of HA helps to keep the plasma proteins in the blood vessel rather than allowing them to enter into the matrix. It also maintains the viscosity of the crystalline liquid-solid water in the matrix and absorbs mechanical and electrical shocks by absorbing sudden changes in electrical potential produced by the storage, uptake, and release of electrons. Hyaluronins affect the solubility of the fibers in the ECM and stabilize the structure of collagens. They also influence matrix chemistry and the binding proteins on cell surfaces that connect molecules.

In the synovial membranes of joints and other organs that have moving surfaces (lungs, heart, joints), the hyaluronin-proteoglycan complex forms the basic lubricant—synovial fluid—that keeps the surfaces slick and moving. The cartilage covered by this material includes the even more slippery sulfated GAGs like chondroitin sulfate; it is slicker than a newly smoothed-over ice rink. This fact has practical pathological significance.

The common denominator of the highly etiologically-variable diseases of the rheumatic type thus lies in pathological changes in the hyaluronic acid and the proteoglycans bound to it. (Pischinger 1991, citing earlier sources)

What this means is that all the different kinds of rheumatic and arthritic diseases, with their different origins—with the exception of autoimmune disease—can be reduced largely to a single origin in the PG/HA "feathers" of the matrix. This is good news from the standpoint of holistic treatment, since we don't need to treat the many different diseases of this kind with different agents, but with one basic theory and a few basic remedies. These types of diseases may also be indicative of a more general lack of HA in the body that needs remedial attention.

HA can expand or contract like a sponge, depending on how dry or damp it is. Therefore, it is especially abundant in load-bearing joints and tissues that absorb and release water continuously. It also is predominant in the interstitial gels in the matrix. In a less hydrated state, it coils up along the protein backbone it is attached to, but when fully hydrated, in unfolds and feathers out across the matrix. Clearly, it has a dominant action on the connective tissue system of the organism, and these observations do not even include discussion of the chondroitin sulfate in cartilage and other polymers that make up the harder connective tissues arising out of the ground substance.

ஒ Mucilaginous Herbal and Food Plants

The importance of HA as a moistening and lubricating substance explains the extremely widespread virtues of mucilaginous medicinal plants like Solomon's Seal (*Polygonatum* spp.), Comfrey (*Symphytum officinale*), and Marshmallow Root (*Althea officinalis*). Mullein (*Verbascum thapsus*) is a salty mucilage that soothes the cilia and linings of the lungs and lubricates joints. Herbalists Sean Donahue and Jim McDonald both encourage the use of Shatavari (*Asparagus racemosus*) as a substitute for Solomon's Seal, which is a wild rather than cultivated plant. Sean wrote to me, "I've seen Shatavari and the roots of garden Asparagus aid synovial fluid in ways similar to, if slightly less pronounced than, Solomon's Seal."

For those who like their mucilage in food, I would recommend Okra (*Abelmoschus esculentus*), a common vegetable in many parts of the world, including the American South. It is quite delicious and should be eaten by people in the North as well, since it is easy to grow and has a short growing season suitable to northern gardens.

Okra is a nice memory from my childhood. My dad came from

Kansas and introduced it to my Brooklyn-born mother. She grew it in the garden; I'm not sure we could have bought it in a store in Minnesota in those days. During the recent food hoarding brought on in the wake of the coronavirus, I noticed that Okra was sometimes the only vegetable left in the freezers in the stores. Don't forget this vegetable, northerners.

Another mucilage that comes up, botanically and gastronomically, but this time from the Southwest and Mexico, is Prickly Pear (*Opuntia* spp.). The pads are filleted and eaten or used as a highly mucilaginous medicine. This tough cactus grows as far north and east as Duluth, Minnesota, though it doesn't get very big. It will be described in more detail in the next chapter.

Increasing Secretion in the Synovia

In addition to increasing the amount and quality of the fluids and the lubricating substances of the matrix, another approach involves opening up the pores of the membranes to allow greater secretion of mucin or the still-more-refined synovial fluid onto mucosal and synovial membranes. The bitters as a whole have a reputation for increasing secretion from the mucosa and internal membranes and structures, but here I will stick (no pun intended) with the remedies that have an established reputation for increasing secretion from these membranes. Perhaps more can be added to this list by future herbal explorers.

The pleura are synovial membranes that lubricate the movement of the lungs and other parts of the body. When the pleura are dried out, adhesions will form where the membranes are stuck together, and when they are dry *and* inflamed, it will become painful to move the membranes. This gives rise to pleurisy in the lungs, pericarditis around the heart, and bursitis in the joints.

❧ *Asclepias tuberosa* (Pleurisy Root)

This is a grand old remedy in American herbalism. It is a native of the continent that received its name somewhere in the dim mists of the eighteenth century, when pleurisy—a harbinger of pneumonia—often meant prolonged illness or death. It was probably introduced from Native American medicine, but the mists of time obscure its history.

Pleurisy Root can also be used for the joints. I have repeatedly seen it remove the adhesions that cause clicking noises as the joints move. Herbalist Jen Tucker uses it for frozen shoulder. It is also useful for congestion and pain in the heart region. I don't know of anyone who has used it for pericarditis, but in conditions that might precede this, where it feels stuffy in the heart region, this herb has repeatedly shown its usefulness. This application was first pointed out by a Muskogee medicine man. He said, "I don't like to talk about this medicine because there will usually be someone in the class who needs it for stuffiness in the chest," and sure enough, there was.

Asclepias does not contain much mucilage, though there is some. It acts more by opening the pores of the skin in fevers and dry persons, and this we see as its operative principle: it opens the pores of the lungs as well as the skin and probably other internal tissues as well. In a typical case, the top of the lungs is more likely to be dry while the bottom is damp, as if the fluids had lost their buoyancy and succumbed to gravity. The pulse has an obstructed feeling in some cases. The milkweed-like seedpod looks like a lung opening up.

ê❧ *Bryonia alba* (White Briony, Mandrake)

This is the homeopathic remedy for pleurisy and pericarditis: indicated when the surfaces are intensely hot and dry, making movement worse. These people don't click and clack when they move; they don't want to move because movement is so painful. This gives rise to the characteristic homeopathic symptom: "worse from movement." Usually, the internal membranes are very hot and dry, the tongue deep red and dried out.

Bryonia is generally suited to acute conditions that come on suddenly. The serous fluids from the capillaries and the matrix provide the lubrication between the sheaths of muscles, so this is also a remedy for pain in the muscles. *Asclepias,* by comparison, is better suited to long-term damage from lingering problems, though it was widely used in the old days for myriads of different kinds of fever in which the skin was dry.

Bryonia was called Mandrake in British herbalism and served a very important purpose. It is a powerful cathartic that must be diluted in order to be used safely. Methods of preparation for safe use were held in secret by the herb guilds that regulated the trade in the countryside and it was used as a symbol by herbalists who held guild status.

Hyaluronidase

Some bacteria and cancer cells generate—and many snake venoms also contain—hyaluronidase, the enzyme mentioned above that dissolves HA, allowing disease processes to spread in the organism. Echinacea, the original "snake oil," contains an antidote to hyaluronidase. It is therefore an ideal remedy for snakebites and pus-producing bacterial infections that contain this enzyme, which is used to spread their deleterious influence through the matrix. In may also have an effect on cancer.

ह≫ *Echinacea* spp.

Dr. H. C. Meyer was a frontier doctor in Pawnee City, Nebraska, in the 1870s, who was friendly with the recently defeated and reservation-bound Lakota people in the western Dakota Territory. From them, he heard about a medicine for snakebite, and finding that it was beneficial, he would sell it and they would pick it for him. The doctor would go to county and state fairs with rattlesnakes penned up in a cage. He would boast to crowds that if he let the snake bite his arm, he would not die because of his medicine. After being bitten in front of astonished crowds, he applied his famous "snake oil." Meyer became a millionaire, and the Lakota people made a share of that money.

After he had made his millions and wanted to retire, Meyer requested that the Eclectic Medical Institute in Cleveland, the foremost school of botanical medicine, identify the plant, which was a secret even to him. He sent a sample to John Uri Lloyd, the great botanical pharmacist, but he was loath to get involved with a man dismissed as a "snake oil salesman" (indeed, the originator of the name). However, Dr. John King, a prominent eclectic medical doctor, had an immediate need for the remedy. His wife had a slowly infiltrating cancer that was very painful, and King wanted to make her more comfortable. He found that Echinacea was very helpful in promoting comfort. She eventually died of the cancer, but King was grateful for the relief it had brought her, and Lloyd was, as he would always report, chastened by the experience. The plant was identified as *Echinacea angustifolia.*

Echinacea became identified with the eclectic medical movement to the extent that it was actively denounced by the American Medical Association. However, many doctors in the rattlesnake-infested regions of the American South and West used it as a reliable antidote. It is much cheaper than the modern pharmaceutical antidote, but neither one is entirely reliable.

In the arrogance typical of science, the highly successful empirical remedy, the "snake oil," was parodied and dismissed by the medical profession and replaced by a pharmaceutical drug that, last time I checked, cost $45,000 per treatment.

Folk medicine is not treated with such contempt in Germany. In the 1930s, a group of German botanical pharmacologists paid a friendly visit to the Eclectic Medical Institute and the Lloyd Brothers Pharmacy. Lloyd was world famous. They wanted to know what particular medicinal plants the Americans knew about that would make a good addition to German botanical medicine. This is when European pharmaceutical companies were first introduced to Echinacea. However, they did make a switch: it was a lot easier to grow *Echinacea purpurea* (Eastern Coneflower) in Europe than to obtain the wild

E. angustifolia traditionally used in American herbalism. It is generally thought that the *E. angustifolia* is superior to the *E. purpurea;* at least it has a larger root. Today, a half dozen *Echinacea* species are used fairly interchangeably.

There is a history of the use of Eastern Coneflower for rattlesnake bite. In the 1750s, an enslaved root doctor named Sampson was given £100 and his freedom by the legislature of South Carolina for revealing his snakebite remedy: *Echinacea purpurea,* also called Black Sampson Root.

Chondroitin Sulfate

This is the most numerous sulfated GAG; it enters into the production of cartilage, tendon, ligament, and bone and is responsible for most of the resistance to compression in structural tissue. It is closely related to HA in structure and is frequently associated with it in cartilage and connective tissues. This suggests that a high priority for ancient lifeforms was protection against the buffeting of the environment of the ocean. It is located primarily in cartilage and at the calcification sites in the bone, but it also occurs in malignant growths, and it is believed to be active in attempting to control aberrant cells from spreading.

ॐ *Eupatorium perfoliatum* (Boneset)

Although I am not sure that Boneset has a specific relationship to chondroitin, it is rather specific in bone injuries where there has been breakage, crushing, or compression. It was not supposed to be a bone-healing remedy, according to a White know-it-all professor in the nineteenth century who stated this as a fact, but it is known as a bone-setting remedy among Native people living within its range, and the name undoubtedly comes from this practice. Our Muskogee teacher called it "Bonemend," and when I asked a member of the Warren family at White Earth, a reservation in northern Minnesota, what was the meaning of its Ojibwa name, he said, "Bone, to mend." Another Ojibwa, Keewaydinoquay, used it for herself and others for bone healing. Herbalist Phyllis Light, of Arab, Alabama, learned of its use from her Creek grandmother, who was a well-known herbalist in that area. This tradition was confirmed by the late Rosalie Wahl, a Minnesota Supreme Court justice who grew up on the Kansas-Oklahoma line and was a close friend of my family.

I first heard about bone healing with Boneset from a woman who lived out near me when I lived at Sunnyfield Herb Farm, in Minnetrista, Minnesota. She had a compression fracture of the carpals in both hands from a car accident and had also lost her two front teeth. The paramedics put the teeth back in, saying "sometimes" they grow back. She took Boneset tea, and her hands and teeth entirely healed. That means the Boneset acted on the tendons holding the teeth to the bone. She loved the taste of the tea, which most people hate.

My favorite case, however, was that of a student who had been so inspired by my herb classes that he decided to go to acupuncture school and make it his profession. However, I got a call the next December. He was miserable, dispirited—I darn say, crushed. He had fallen flat on his back on the sheet ice in a parking lot and was confined to bed, where he was in great pain. There were no broken bones, but the injury was diagnosed as a widespread compression injury of the spinal vertebra. Boneset had him cheered up and back on his feet in a few days. He came by to personally thank me.

Since all the connective tissues arise from similar, related cells (fibroblasts or modified versions thereof), this remedy, like others, seems to act on the connective tissues of the whole system, including cartilage, bone, tendon, and ligament. Probably also on the matrix itself. In fact, it seems to have an ability to expel foreign materials from the matrix and is somewhat antivenomous (Native tradition) and antibacterial (clinical experience).

Heparan Sulfate/Heparin

The next most important GAG in the regulation of the matrix is heparan sulfate. It is made in the Golgi apparatus by the same enzymes as heparin and is similar in structure and function, so the two are discussed and classified together. Heparin is the substance used by doctors to thin the blood (make blood cells less adhesive), but this familiar activity is only one of dozens of functions of heparin and should not be looked on as the most important.

Both heparan sulfate and heparin, after manufacture in the Golgi apparatus, are moved in vacuoles to the surface of the cell membrane, from whence they begin their travels and functions. They are both composed of disaccharide units—less in heparan sulfate, more in heparin. However, there are hybrids between the two, so these two polymers must be looked on as lying on a continuum rather than constituting completely unrelated articles. This is in part due to the fact that they are made in many different kinds of cells to fulfill many different functions. The main difference is that heparin is free circulating while heparan sulfate is usually tightly bound to the cell membrane. These locations relate to the separate but often analogous functions of the two. In conformity with scientific usage we can discuss them, in some cases, as though they are one entity: heparan sulfate/heparin (HS/H).

HS/H is active in every known element of regulation that occurs in the matrix. It operates on and modifies many of the activities of HA and the cells. It influences the breakdown of the fatty end of lipoproteins (cholesterol) in the circulating blood by activating the necessary enzyme for lipolysis in the endothelium of the blood vessel. This is an all-important function from the standpoint of vascular health. It is also involved in the synthesis of fibroblasts, so it has an influence on the hyaluronins and other GAGs available to plump up the ECM. It also acts on the fibers once they have been manufactured and extruded into the matrix. HS/H is involved in the activation of no less than fifty different enzymes, involving numerous processes in the matrix and elsewhere, including immune tolerance, recovery from anaphylaxis, and angiogenesis—the generation of new blood vessels from old. Some HS/H remains in the cell and interacts with the transcription of the all-important DNA and RNA proteins inside the cell.

HS/H is stored in mast cells, a type of white blood cell that also contains histamines active in the inflammatory response. Best known for their activity in allergic and anaphylaxis responses, histamines are also involved in wound healing, angiogenesis, immune tolerance, the blood-brain barrier, and defense against pathogens. Angiogenesis reduces inflammation because the generation of new and additional blood vessels spreads out the blood, gives the heat in it greater access to the surface for discharge, and is therefore cooling. Angiogenesis is a property attributed to Lavender by Dietrich Gümbel in *Principles of Holistic Therapy with Herbal Essences* (1993).

Mast cells are capable of movement and travel toward autonomic nerve tissues. Since these tissues are found in close proximity to the capillary bed and larger blood vessels, this is where the mast cells congregate. In other words, they are stationed perfectly to meet with allergens and bacteria that are coming in through the capillary bed.

When the catecholamines epinephrine (adrenaline), norepinephrine (noradrenaline), and dopamine are released by the adrenal medulla and other tissues in the fight-or-flight response, they travel to the capillary bed and are diffused into the matrix, triggering the release of histamine and heparin granules stored in the cell. The "adrenaline response" extends all the way to the matrix. Other factors, such as changes toward an acid pH, allergy, leukotriene increase, and many more, can initiate the unloading of histamines and HS/H from the mast cells.

Heparan sulfate is a linear polymer (unlike the coiled HA) that usually bonds with the cell membrane as it is extruded from the vacuole through the membrane. Unlike the other GAGs, it binds to a proteoglycan that is hydrophobic, so it does not absorb or mix with water but rather bonds strongly to the lipophilic cell membrane and cannot be separated except by *lysis* (breakdown) of the protein connector. It contributes to cell adhesiveness, regulates cell growth and proliferation and cellular developmental processes, and protects from viral invasion, blood coagulation, and tumor metastasis. It has a protective effect against some viruses. It also helps bind cells to the basement membrane and has an influence on cell reproduction and differentiation.

Although heparan sulfate adheres to cells, heparin circulates freely in the blood and serum. It thins the blood by decreasing the adhesiveness of blood cells to one another, therefore preventing them from clumping and clotting. It also inhibits one of the factors in the chain reaction that creates clots. This is why it is used as a blood thinner in medicine. However, "The coagulation-inhibiting function of heparin is wrongly placed in the foreground," writes Pischinger (1991, 47). As with sulfation factor, I was astonished when I learned about the greater complexity and scope of activities of HS/H. Once again, we are reminded of the importance of perspective. Research has shown that nebulized heparin can be an extremely supportive anti-coagulative therapy for badly damaged lung tissue (Juschten et al. 2017).

Keratan Sulfate

This GAG affects cell adhesion, including macrophage adhesion, and assists with immune reaction, embryo implantation in the endometrium of the uterus, and motility of corneal endothelial cells. Maintenance of tissue hydration is another major function of keratan sulfate.

The relationship of keratan sulfate to the cornea has been known for a long time. Within the healthy cornea, dermatan sulfate is fully hydrated, whereas keratan sulfate is only partly hydrated. Some suggest that the latter buffers hydration. There is a long-held hypothesis that cataracts are due to improper levels of keratan sulfate.

﷼ Bilberry (*Vaccinium myrtillus*)

This is the most famous eye-specific medicine plant. Bilberries have been eaten and used as medicines from time immemorial, but they rose to fame during World War II, when British pilots supposedly ate bilberry jam with the belief that it increased their night vision. It has since been found to be beneficial in practice for various eye problems, even to remove cataracts. My friend Paul Red Elk said that his grandfather, a traditional medicine man on the Rosebud reservation in South Dakota, used this herb, which was introduced from Europe. He called it "Bright Bill."

Not only is Bilberry an astringent, it also reduces autoimmune excess, so that it almost certainly acts on the mast cell functions listed under heparan sulfate. The connection between cataracts and keratan sulfate reminded me of something I have sometimes observed in people with eye problems. They often respond very well to astringents, which are in fact remedies that encourage drying. Others need the moistening mucilages.

Bilberry is a close relative of Blueberry and Huckleberry (*Vaccinium* spp.) but is native to Europe, while they are native to America. It contains a higher level of the so-called active ingredients—anthocyanins—that are cooling and sedative to the immune system. It is also an astringent (a property overlooked in the scientific literature for the most part, but very important). It is more tart than a blueberry but has a similar taste. As an eye remedy, it has assumed a profile all its own.

Bilberries were traditionally used for scurvy (they contain plenty of vitamin C), diarrhea (astringent), infections and burns (cooling, antiseptic, like many members of the Heath family), and diabetes. Both Blueberry and Bilberry are old folk remedies for type 2 diabetes, each in a different part of the world, so this testifies to a reliable medicinal effect. Bilberries contain more anthocyanins than Blueberry; these are sedating to an overactive immune system. The high level of anthocyanins gives the Bilberry a darker color than its cousin. Blueberry leaves are used to curtail excessive urination in people with diabetes. Today, Bilberry is used for cardiovascular conditions (cooling to the capillaries, mast cells, heparan), urinary tract infections (almost every Heath family plant is used for this), eye problems, and diabetes or high blood sugar. The Commission E scientific advisory board in Germany has approved its use for inflammation of the mouth and intestines, with diarrhea.

I have not used this plant a lot, but I have noticed that it sometimes changes the circulation from the brain going toward the eyes and nose.

A scientific roundup of materials on Bilberry can be found in the review "Bilberry (*Vaccinium myrtillus* L.)" in the book *Herbal Medicine: Biomolecular and Clinical Aspects* (Chu et al. 2011).

Dermatan Sulfate

This GAG increases structural integrity in many tissues. It reinforces the skin and helps with wound healing. It contributes to the integrity of the cornea and sclera of the eye, maintaining the shape of the eye and the transparency of the cornea necessary for visual acuity. It is also found in cartilage and bone tissue (combined with chondroitin sulfate). As a structural element, it contributes to the strength of blood vessels, heart valves, and the umbilical cord. It also decreases the coagulability of the blood. It may inhibit the formation of atherosclerosis. In addition, dermatan sulfate interacts with matrix proteins, lipoproteins, growth factors, cytokines, and cell surface receptors. It is believed to have an influence on cellular proliferation (by interacting with fibroblast growth factor). It also is believed to influence the defense against pathogens and inflammation and inhibit the development of cancer.

Dermatan sulfate interacts with chondroitin sulfate and ought to have some affinity to the same medicinal agents, mostly mucilages, mentioned in the discussion of GAGs.

PROTEOGLYCANS (PGS)

Now that we have discussed the GAGs, we can move to the structures built from them, the proteoglycans. PGs provide structure, strength, padding, and flexibility. Some are flexible, pulpy, and elastic, while others are stronger than steel and more adherent than anything made by the hand of man. For instance, the glue that holds barnacles onto ships is a type of matrix polymer that is stronger than any known man-made adhesive. PGs also transmit signals through changes in electric potential. Through a mixture of mechanical properties and signals, they condition and control the environment of the cells.

The appropriate level of an ion in the ECF is called the "isotonic balance." PGs guarantee this balance, which in turn modifies the isoosmic balance (osmotic pressure), in the matrix. These isotonic processes regulate the tension in the PGs and fibers themselves.

PGs have all sorts of connections to the immune system. They are capable of disrupting most, possibly all, key steps in the genesis of microbial disease in the body. This includes initial invasion, dissemination and infection to secondary locations, microbial attachment to cells in the body, and evasion of host defense mechanisms; they also heighten cell-to-cell transmission of immune information. PGs also help control the spread of toxins, either those that enter from the outside or those generated within the organism.

Proteoglycans always remain inside the matrix in the lower life-forms, but in higher animal life-forms some of them are secreted into body cavities and surfaces to thicken water into glairy fluids like mucin and synovial fluid. The spermatic fluid carrying gamete cells is composed of PGs, and the walls of the fallopian tubes and uterus are coated with the PG mucin. Reproduction in higher animals depends on healthy matrix polymers. The emphasis on hormone balancing alone in modern fertility clinics represents incomplete thinking: if a man or woman does not have good PGs, he or she will be infertile. In other cases there is an excess of mucin. Other factors are a lack of good quality lipids to make good hormones and the ability to digest them or process them in the liver. Numerous herbalists, including myself, have brought about the desired pregnancy through the use of herbs addressing these issues. Easter Lily (*Lilium longiflorum*) is an excellent remedy for adjusting mucin levels in the fallopian tubes and uterus and is often used to treat infertility.

In the last several decades, PGs have become widely used as supplements. Commercial glucosamine sulfate is a mix of PGs and

GAGs derived from calf trachea (a by-product of the veal industry). It is about 70 percent absorbable across the intestinal membrane. Chondroitin sulfate is derived from shark cartilage (a byproduct of the fishing industry). It is less than 10 percent absorbable through the gut wall, so a modified form, chondroitin hydrochloride, has been introduced.

CONNECTIVE TISSUE CELLS

The original fibroblasts generate GAGs differentiated into chrondroblasts (cartilage-generating), tenocytes (tendon-making), and osteoblasts (bone-making). All together, these compose the connective tissue cells and are the progenitors of the connective tissue system— one of the four primal systems of the body. They are matched by the chrondroclasts, tendinoclasts, and osteoclasts that break these materials down.

Fibroblasts

In order to produce the polymers and fibers of the matrix more efficiently, cells evolved into fibroblasts, which specialize in these activities. Fibroblasts react immediately to a great variety of incoming information from hormones, neurotransmitters, catabolites, anabolites, pH, and such. In response, they metabolize the materials necessary to maintain the matrix. They do not differentiate between healthy and unhealthy information. This is of great importance in the modern world, where human beings have damaged not just the external environment but the internal as well.

Fibroblasts are covered by a coating that is partly constructed of HA, which protects them from bacteria and various foreign molecules in the matrix. Hyaluronins, with chondroitin sulfate, help form a structural niche within which sits the fibroblast stem cell. This protects it from growth factors that would alter the identity of the stem cell. During cell division, the daughter cell moves outside this shield so it can be influenced by growth factors that determine what it is to become. In this way, the stem cells in the bone marrow produce new red blood cells, white blood cells, and replacement parts for the rest of the body. (This is why blood is classified as a connective tissue.) If the daughter cells are not protected, they can become defective, die, not undertake their correct function, or generate cancer.

ॐ Calcium Phosphate

There are many uses of calcium phosphate that are very important when it is given as a physical supplement or in the form of a homeopathic remedy. However, one that is overlooked is the protection of the daughter cells by the connective tissue surrounding them as they are being made. This is particularly easy to visualize when it comes to the bone marrow's production of red cells and white cells. This explains why, as a homeopathic application or a cell salt, calcium phosphate is a remedy for anemia and low immune function. As for regrowth of bone, I have had two clients who regrew two inches they had lost to osteoporosis.

As to the use of calcium supplements, one should be aware that excess calcium causes some of the same problems as a deficiency—most notably, osteoporosis. Problems with calcium can be avoided by the consumption of vitamin K2, which directs the calcium in the appropriate fashion. This vitamin turns out to be the "factor X" that was discovered by Weston Price in the 1930s, but not identified until recently.

Chondroblasts and Cartilage

As higher life-forms developed, fibroblasts moved from the generation of polymers to the manufacture of fibers or chains that were wider than one molecule. This was the origin of the primal fibers or collagens of the structural system of the multicellular organism. The fibroblasts themselves were modified in this transition, becoming the chondroblasts that produce hard, elastic structures to make organisms still more resistant to the environment. These substances comprise the fascia and cartilage that are the basic structural and compartmentalizing materials of the body, as well as the sinews and bones of mobile animal life.

The interior of cartilage is composed of the ground substance of the matrix, which some have likened to the lofty beams of Chartres Cathedral. It is fed and watered by currents moving slowly through it. Cartilage does not possess its own blood supply. The capillaries dump off water, food, oxygen, and other substances at the boundary of the cartilage, inside of which slow-moving currents disseminate them throughout the cartilaginous structure. This is why cartilage is white or pale: it possesses no blood. This is also why cartilaginous injuries are so hard to repair: the tissue is too slowly nourished for regrowth to take place efficiently. The slow, passive currents in the cartilage are generated by movements of the joint, so exercise is helpful in maintaining joint health, unless it is excessive or improper.

ᒥ *Symphytum officinale* (Comfrey Leaf, Root)

This ancient medicinal plant is perfectly suited to the repair of cartilaginous injuries. First, it is an astringent classified as a "drawing agent," so it draws the fluids and their contents through the cartilage. Second, it contains allantoin, a substance that increases growth. Third, as a mucilage, it contains many of the same substances found in cartilage.

The pulling power of Comfrey is very real. I remember hearing at an herbal conference of a case history in which a comfrey poultice on an injured joint started pulling blood through the skin; this warned the client and the herbalist that a visit to the doctor was needed. On the other hand, Comfrey tends to heal from the surface down, rather than from the bottom up, so that it can cause broken bones that are not set right to heal in the wrong places. This is even true of the homeopathic Symphytum, according to Robin Murphy, N.D.

Further Differentiation of Connective Tissue

Cartilage eventually developed through evolution to form sinews, bones, and joints—in short, the structural materials of animals. The cells that produce these structures are tenocytes (sinews) and osteoblasts (bone).

The common origin of these connective tissue cells in fibroblasts is significant from the herbal standpoint because many of the remedies that are well known for healing one connective tissue structure will act on others. Comfrey, Solomon's Seal, Boneset, and probably Marshmallow should all be considered from this perspective.

One would think the best way to make healthy connective tissue would be to increase and support the generation of new tissue (the "blast" side of the equation, as in the job of osteoblasts), but biomedicine is capable only of stopping the breakdown of connective tissue (the job of the osteoclasts). The drug Fosamax kills the osteoclasts so that they cannot break down old, deteriorating bone tissue as they normally would. But, by increasing the amount of old, worn-out tissue, this drug produces side effects such as spontaneous, catastrophic breakage of the hipbones and "dead jaw syndrome." This isn't as bad as it sounds: only the lower jaw is completely destroyed and removed, not the upper jaw as well. This "side-effect" of the drug was discovered by dentists, not medical doctors.

Research has shown that changes in diet and exercise can reverse osteoporosis, and there are many herbs that have proven successful in this regard. My favorite agent is homeopathic Calcium phosphate.

DIFFERENT KINDS OF CONNECTIVE TISSUE FIBER

The fibers of the connective tissue system are specialized proteins generated by the fibroblasts and the cellular "descendants" described above. The main protein fibers of this system are four in number: collagens, elastins, fibronectins, and laminins. Together, they produce the fiber, cartilage, sinews, bones, and joints that provide the body with structure, hardness, leverage, and the ability to move.

Collagen

Fibroblasts manufacture collagens, which constitute the main structural component of the matrix—and of the body as a whole. In the matrix, they provide strength and tension, anchor cells together, regulate cell adhesion, and direct self-development. Not only do the fibroblasts organize collagens into fibrous cables and sheets, they also align these structures.

Within a tissue, there are several different kinds of collagen, and they are organized into a mix of different types, though one is likely to predominate. On the macroscopic level, they figure in the construction of bones, muscles, tendons, and skin. Combined with the microscopic level in the matrix, these different collagens literally hold the body together. They are massive in quantity, composing as much as 30 percent of the total protein mass in a multicellular animal, and are the single most abundant protein.

Collagen is so strong because it is composed of a triple helix of protein strands, not just a double helix, as found in genetic material. Proteins contain more nitrogen than other organic components of the body; this is the element that resists oxidation and therefore retards the weathering, breakdown, and aging of collagens as well as DNAs and RNAs.

Collagen fibers join together to form *microfibrils,* semicrystalline structures of repeating molecules that are conductive and resistant to electrical signals. Microfibrils form along lines of stress in the body to create the structural materials we are familiar with: fascia, cartilage, sinews, and such. Piezoelectricity moves along the microfibrils, regulating and maintaining the health of the larger connective tissue structures.

There are at least sixteen different kinds of collagen—with different structures, functions, and strengths—but 80 to 90 percent of them are classified as collagens I, II, or III. Some kinds are stronger than steel, while others are smoother than ice. Think of the sleek surface of Jell-O (gelatin) or a piece of cartilage taken from the breast of a chicken: gelatin is composed of hydrolyzed collagen. For contrast, think of the concretions holding the barnacle on a boat or rock.

Endogenous collagen is synthesized within the body, while *exogenous collagen* is derived from an external dietary source such as animal connective tissue. All collagen supplements come from animals, since plants cannot produce collagen. These supplements are used in medicine, alternative medicine, and cosmetology. Collagen production declines with age and exposure to factors including smoking and UV light. Collagen molecules are considered to be too large to be absorbed through the skin, but they are used in wound dressings to attract new skin cells to the area.

The manufacture of collagen requires vitamin C. A shortage of this vitamin therefore causes the breakdown of collagen, which results in scurvy, heralded by bleeding from the gums, as the structural material breaks down and cannot be repaired. This gave rise to the use of citrus fruits, high in vitamin C, to prevent scurvy in sailors on long voyages. Since cancer spreads through the fascia, which is composed of collagen, one can see at once the logic of American biochemist Linus Pauling's idea that vitamin C reduces tendencies to cancer. Despite this simple logic, this idea was ignored in conventional biomedicine until the last decade.

Elastin

Elastin fibers provide elasticity and are found in connective tissues that undergo repeated stretching and contraction. The return of skin to normal shape after it has been poked requires healthy elastin in the connective tissue. The stretchability and elasticity of a tissue is limited by the amount of collagens and lysine amino acids present. Elastins are covered by glycoprotein microfibrils, which maintain their integrity.

It is hard to visualize elastins and what they do from the above "fact sheet," but these functions can be translated into simple terms that people can easily understand. When the elastin in a tissue has been damaged in some way, tissues can lose their tone, sag, and even prolapse. To judge from complementary and alternative medicine practices, there are at least three different ways this can occur.

Cell salts teach us that the first problem is nutritional, involving a lack of calcium fluoride or the element fluorine. This element is highly toxic, but is found in small amounts mostly in the teeth (making enamel), the bones, and structures requiring elasticity and stretchability. It seems to act simultaneously to both harden tissue and make it more elastic and less brittle. All of these indications are associated with the cell salt Calcium fluoride.

The second problem seems to be due to the loss of the glycoprotein microfibrils that coat and protect the elastins. This condition is probably directly treatable by the protein tannins in astringents that coat membranes and allow them to tighten and rebuild themselves. It is notable that the range of action of White Oak bark (*Quercus alba*) is very similar to that of Calcium fluoride. The great astringents in addition are Schizandra, Lady's Mantle, Raspberry Leaf and Blackberry root. Sumac (*Rhus* spp.) is an underrated astringent.

The third problem seems to be caused by the flowing off of water from the poorly toned pores in stretchable tissue. Astringents close these pores, but care should be taken not to suppress a discharge. In traditional Chinese herbalism, "yang tonics," or warming agents, are used often instead of astringents. These are called "solar remedies" in Western astrological medicine. They are like sunlight beating on the sidewalk on a hot summer day, vaporizing away the excess water. Examples of herbs with this gentle warming action include Angelica, St. John's Wort, Rosemary, Calendula, Thyme, and Savory.

Fibronectin

A third fibrous protein, fibronectin, helps to direct the organization of the matrix, maintaining the structural stability and functional capacities of important organs and tissues. In addition, it mediates cell attachment and function.

Fibronectin can be stretched several times longer than its normal length at rest by the traction forces of the cells. This exposes hidden binding sites that, when activated, regulate cell function. Fibronectin therefore is important for cell migration during tissue maturation and fibroblast migration to facilitate wound healing. It is also active in the formation of new capillaries (angiogenesis), clot formation, and platelet activity, so it is important in the life of the circulatory system and also the transition to and from scab formation in wound repair. It also assists collagen biosynthesis and epithelial regrowth after injury. Because of their relationship to tension, fibronectins can influence cardiovascular health, and because of their relationship to cell migration, they can influence tumor growth. Altogether, fibronectin is essential for cell migration, proliferation, differentiation, adhesion, signaling, and apoptosis (an internal programming mechanism that brings about the death of old, worn-out cells).

In some ways, fibronectin has an opposite action from elastin: the former stretches, while the latter contracts. I am not clear enough on the pharmacology and botanical medicine of fibronectin to assert any therapeutic ideas with any certainty, but we know in herbalism that the acrid flavor is associated with relaxation. This can be on the physical, psychological, and even the spiritual level since some of the strongest relaxing acrid plant substances are hallucinogenic, including the "spirit molecule," dimethyltryptamine (DMT). The alkaloids as a class are acrid.

If there is a universal remedy for tension and tightness, it is certainly magnesium, an element that is required in order for the tissues to relax and which many people are short on. Among the plant medicines, the most acrid relaxant is Lobelia (*Lobelia inflata*). This remarkable remedy, made known by the backwoods New Hampshire farmer Samuel Thomson (1769–1843), is often too active for use and requires a special hand for intelligent use. Nigella Seed (*Nigella sativa*) is a milder acrid relaxant with similar properties; I call it "Lobelia's little brother." In addition, it has innumerable immune-stimulating and other properties.

Laminins

These proteogylcans compose an important part of the basal lamina, a layer in the basement membrane separating the matrix from various tissues and organs, and form part of the structural scaffolding supporting almost every tissue in the body. They also influence cell differentiation, migration, and adhesion. Although less common than the other fibers, laminin is vital for tissue health. It is found in peripheral nerves, dorsal root ganglions, skeletal muscle, neuromuscular junctions, and the capillaries of the blood, so it is associated with one kind of muscular dystrophy, the blood-filtering mechanism in the kidneys, and other rare and lethal diseases. One thing I know for sure from treating horses and people: Dandelion root usually stops inflammation in bones and lamina.

THE COMPLETE ECM

Altogether, the components of the matrix have been completely cataloged now. They are sometimes classified into two groups (Alfano et al. 2016):

1. *Macromolecules:* consisting of the matrisomes, 43 collagen subunits, and 35 proteoglycans, and
2. *Matrisome-associated molecules:* including 250 matrix regulators, 176 matrix-affiliated proteins, and 352 secreted factors bound to the matrix, such as matrix metalloproteinases, metalloproteinase inhibitors, mucins, and TGF-β (a transforming growth factor).

This tabulation does not include the fibroblasts, macrophages, mast cells, and other immune cells. The usual boundary line is set between the ground substance and the cell, although these cells serve the matrix. These cells will be discussed with other cells in chapter 5.

The exact numbers provided above might mislead us. We should not imagine a stationary ECM. The matrix is constantly changing composition, shape, strength, and so on. The blood and lymphatic capillaries that interpenetrate the matrix are themselves constantly developing new vessels, locations, and shapes. The structure of the ECM changes in different tissues and organs, and the stiffness and shapes of extracellular spaces function to modify cell phenotypes and the function of the cells and organs. Even the type of cells drawn in from the circulation can differ from tissue to tissue, or organ to organ, due to the differing composition of the matrix. The fate of these incoming cells and their differentiation and applications are also modified by the matrix according to region.

> All the tissues of the body are in a state of ebb and flow. Where life is there is no standing still; everything is in a state of motion and change. The tissues once built up from the food no sooner reach their perfection and perform their function than they begin to decay and make room for more. Some tissues change more rapidly than others—the soft tissues more rapidly than the hard—but all change and break down into their elements. (Clarke 1886)

BACTERIA AND THE MATRIX

Hardly has the paint dried on the knowledge of the ECM and the GRS when a new signaling method has been discovered that is used by bacteria. This can cause groups of bacteria to work together as a united community toward a common goal. It works both inside the matrix and in the microbiome living on the outside of the matrix. This information is quite new and probably incomplete. It is possible that cells in the organism use a similar method.

Communication between bacteria of the same or different species relies on signaling molecules called *autoinducers*. These signals cause changes in gene expression in the bacteria, and this changes their behavior, including reproduction. This form of communication is called *quorum sensing* because the signals start really "talking" when they reach a quorum or critical mass.

Individual bacteria generate autoinducers during their reproductive cycle. Gram-negative bacteria produce ones that passively diffuse through the cell membranes, while gram-positive bacteria produce others that have to be actively transported across the membrane. Both use a transporter system that relies on an aspect of the ATP cycle (see chapter 5) that brings energy from mitochondria to the cell membrane for energy shortage. This means that energy for living and signals for communication depend on a healthy level of mitochondrial function and cell membrane integrity.

As long as the bacteria are reproducing, their numbers are increasing, more autoinducers are being synthesized, and more are migrating out into the matrix. When the autoinducers' numbers inside and out become about even, they stop moving out of the cells. At this point, they are inhibited from leaving the cells by the transcription factors that control their gene expression. This is the quorum that causes the signaling shift. The increased intracellular concentration causes the autoinducers to bind to their receptor sites in other cells, triggering signaling cascades that cause new alterations in transcription factors and subsequent gene expression. This "allows individual bacteria within colonies to coordinate and carry out colony-wide functions such as: sporulation, bioluminescence, virulence, conjugation, competence and biofilm formation" (Windsor 2020). This can enable bacteria to quickly increase in virulence and biofilm manufacturing.

Not only do bacteria within a species communicate by quorum sensing, interspecies quorum sensing also occurs, causing both competition and collaboration. One species can make another more virulent, but we can also benefit from quorum sensing. The so-called friendly bacteria living symbiotically in our intestines can actually control unfriendly competition through quorum sensing. "Like humans, bacteria operate on a continuum of individualism and collectivism" (Windsor 2020).

THE EXTRACELLULAR MATRIX AND THE CONNECTIVE TISSUE SYSTEM

The extracellular matrix is the original, primal organ system of the multicellular organism. The next to arise was the connective tissue system, which is the basis of hardness, stretchiness, protection, compartmentalization, and structure. Through the leverage provided by the hard parts, it sets the stage for movement.

The same materials are found in both the matrix and connective tissue, but in reverse amounts. The ECM is about 70 percent liquid and 30 percent solid, while the connective tissue structures are about 30 percent liquid and 70 percent solid. The development of the structural system out of the matrix was like the rising of a continent out of the ocean.

The first connective tissue consisted of fibers randomly lacing together the amorphous matrix of primitive sea creatures such as jellyfishes. Later, fibroblasts developed the ability to align collagen fibers into sheets and cables to strengthen and harden areas of the organism. They do this by exerting tension against certain regions of the matrix. The collagens combine with elastins to make tissue that varies in hardness and flexibility. Think of the starfish.

The development of subsequent organ systems depended on these two original systems because the organs developed in their own isolated matrices, surrounded by connective tissue. Variations in tension and rest between the different regions of the organism created these spaces. The fact that all tissues, organs, and systems developed out of these two primal systems reminds us how important they are and how we must learn to heal them in order to assist all regions, systems, and functions in the body.

Fascia

The first organized connective tissue structure is the *fascia*. The word derives from the Latin, meaning "bands," and it is still used in the building industry to designate pieces that connect one part to another. Ignored until the last decade, the fascia in our bodies is now a sort of darling of medical research; this is also a connective point between modern biomedicine, acupuncture, and other forms of traditional medicine. Among the leading names in the study of fascia in complementary and alternative medicine are Gil Hedley and John Barnes.

Fascia is made from the collagen generated by fibroblasts. They intertwine or inter-twirl to create triple helix proteins that recombine again to produce the microfibrils that form fascia. These structures by themselves are thin and nearly transparent but incredibly strong. They are impenetrable and impermeable to water, air, blood, pus, and even electricity, yet they carry electrical charges. They generate an electrical charge when they move, making the fascia composed of them both conductive and resistant to electric currents, like a copper wire. Mention has already been made of this organic charge, called piezoelectricity.

Perhaps more remarkably, fascial tubules contain light, like a fiber optic thread, which, it would seem, brings light deeper into the interior of the body than would otherwise be possible. We remember the importance of sunlight in generating the organic water of life, as discovered by Gerald Pollack.

The fascia makes up the compartments we have been describing above. Every tendon, ligament, bone, nerve, muscle, blood vessel, and organ is covered in fascia. It has no form of its own but allows the development of the form of the tissue or organ developing within it. Daniel Keown (2014, 11) describes the organs as "vacuum-packed in fascia." It even looks a lot like plastic food wrap. It creates separate compartments, yet is never less than contiguous, forming a membrane that is present from head to toe.

Fascia is the primal or original tissue of the connective tissue system as a whole. It also is closely interactive with the matrix from which it arose. However, fascia is also interlaced with tissues that developed later in evolution, such as bones, endocrine glands, immune cells, blood vessels, lymphatic drains, and nerves. The fascia acts, therefore, as a sort of "translator" from the GRS to the higher organism.

The major pathological problems associated with the fascia in conventional biomedicine are inflammation (fasciitis) and "compartment syndrome," in which the fascia tightens up around an inflamed area and can "throttle" the contents, as Keown (2014, 10) colorfully observes. This contributes to pain. There is also the problem that cancer spreads through the fascia.

Keown argues that the "three burning spaces" or "triple heater" of traditional and ancient Chinese medicine are equivalent to the fascia. Both ancient Chinese and modern medicine divide the animal trunk into three functional units, the thoracic, abdominal, and pelvic compartments, which are separated and enclosed by thick fascial envelopments. The lesser and more far-flung fascial tissues are, in a sense, the appendages or extensions of these three core spaces.

The function of the three burning spaces in Chinese medicine is to regulate heat and water, distributing them evenly and smoothly throughout the organism. I would associate these processes with the matrix, with the fascia acting as the "translator" to the rest of the organism. The two are intimately related: the continent of the connective tissue rising up from the sea of the matrix through the fascia and then moving to the more articulated structures.

It is believed that, through deformations caused by injuries, diseases, and emotional upsets, the fascia are marked and twisted into subtle new shapes that hold the memory of the events the organism has suffered. Acupuncture, bodywork, herbs, and flower essences all work on the body memory, removing old deformations and returning to old patterns of health or generating new ones. Thus, the fascia does have a central and important role to play in health, disease, and healing, as visualized by Keown, Hedley, Barnes, and others. It perhaps acts as the translator between the matrix found in primitive multicellular organs and the higher functions and organs later developed.

THE PROBLEM OF THE INTERSTITIUM

On March 27, 2018, *Scientific American* startled the world by announcing the existence of a "newfound 'organ'" called the interstitium (Rettner 2018). Students, researchers, and practitioners in the alternative medicine world who were familiar with the matrix and the fascia were surprised since this clearly described a part of the ECM or the fascia or both—depending on where the lines are drawn—with which they had long been familiar. Scientists and medical doctors of the old school were equally shocked. The interstitium seemed to be new only in the eyes of its discoverers. This was quite an awkward finding.

Tom Myers, an important writer and author on the fascia, responded with a statement that was published two days later at the Anatomy Trains website (Myers 2018). The use of new confocal laser microscopy showed the existence of a tissue that was crushed when conventional microscope slide and staining methods were used. Myers responds to the discovery:

> This tissue system was originally filmed in vivo and described in a number of papers and books by French surgeon Dr. Jean-Claude Guimberteau, described on YouTube by Gil Hedley as peri-fascial membranes, and written about by me in *Anatomy Trains*. (Myers 2018)

Myers notes that even among these three individuals, the interstitium went by three separate names: "fascia" (Myers), "peri-fascial membranes" (Hedley), and "microvacuolar system" (Guimberteau).

So what is the interstitium? It is a "bubbly gel" located between layers of more dense fascia. It is also composed of collagen and elastin fibers suspended in interstitial fluids (hence the name interstitium). Older imaging suggested that this area was filled with hard fascia, but new instrumentation showed that this humid, bubbly gel contains up to one-third of the fluid of the body at any given moment.

The interstitium possesses three major mechanical properties: viscosity, elasticity, and plasticity. The first dissipates sudden concentrations of force so that it acts effectively like padding between fascial layers. The elasticity allows changes of shape that return to normal after temporary forces return to rest. The plasticity encourages remodeling of deformations caused by long-term stresses such as aging, injury, scarring, and even change of occupation. Thus, it provides the "context for all movement," states Myers, yet it transcends even this noble function for it acts as a continuous "biomechanical auto-regulatory system" (Myers 2018). The interstitium receives signals that move from the DNA in the cell through the cell and cell surface to the polymers of the GRS, and thence to the fascia. From there, signals move out to the sinews, bones, joints, muscles, and the entire locomotor system. The interstitium is frequently aligned with lymphatic ducts, so it also is intimate with white blood cells and immune signals. So the interstitium is the "translator" from the deepest interior and the middle ground of the body all the way out to the organs of transportation in the physical environment. Through movement, repetition, and injury, it receives signals from the environment and surface that travel back the other way, into the middle ground and interior reaches of the body. It also interacts with cognitive signals that control movement and with unconscious ones in the autonomic nervous system that support movement. One can see how it becomes a storehouse for body memory.

Another important point about the interstitium is that it is believed that certain cancers travel through it. We know that cancers use the GRS. They move from the matrix, sometimes, to the interstitium and thence through the fascia, which means they are "spreading."

Myers concludes:

That these scientists have imaged something they missed for years is great, but the larger insight is that our "biomechanics"—muscles work via tendons over joints restrained by ligaments—requires total re-think in terms of these new findings of mechanical continuity from molecular on up through cells, tissues, and the entire human being. (Myers 2018)

One can see why scientists thought they had discovered an entirely new "system." However, alternative researchers in fascia—Hedley, Barnes, Myers, and Guimberteau, who first drew attention to this tissue and its importance—had been there first. This is another example of how the intuitive, experiential view, based on the behavior of phenomena, anticipates conventional discoveries and is not acknowledged within the mainstream.

CANCER AND THE MATRIX

As in biomedicine, practitioners of complementary and alternative modalities must specialize, and cancer is not an area that I have specialized in. Looking back, I feel that this was appropriate and fortunate. So many factors enter into the cancer equation that it constitutes a subject worthy of lengthy study. Many of these factors were unknown until the matrix was understood, so it would have been impossible to have a competent overview until after the turn of the millennium.

In 1988, Barbara A. Israel and Warren I. Schaeffer reported the results of research showing that it is the cell membrane that usually determines whether the cell turns cancerous, not the nucleus.

The relative roles of nucleus and cytoplasm in the induction and maintenance of the malignant state were studied. Cytoplasmic hybrid (cybrid) clones, derived from the fusion of cytoplasts from malignantly transformed cells to normal whole cells, produced tumors in 17% of the animals injected with them. Nuclear/cytoplasmic hybrid (reconstituted cell) clones, derived by fusion of cytoplasts from malignant cells with karyoplasts of normal cells, produced tumors in 97% of the animals injected. (Israel and Schaeffer 1988)

In order to treat cancer, we need to visualize it correctly. Although it is a disease of genetic mutation, this study makes clear that it is the cell membrane that is predominately responsible for the shift from normalcy to malignancy. It would be better to see cancer as a disease of signaling, in many cases, rather than of genetic mutation. Cancer arises as a disconnect between the GRS, which keeps all the cells working together harmoniously, and a cell that "wants to go its own way." The cell membrane is the part that is responsible for keeping in touch with the GRS, so this is where the rift between them usually takes place. Additional research shows that malignant cells continue to use signals from the GRS to feed, eliminate, reproduce, and migrate—just as healthy cells do.

In 2000, Hanahan and Weinberg wrestled "the dense complexities of cancer biology" into six basic "hallmarks": "self-sufficiency in growth signals, insensitivity to anti-growth signals, evading apoptosis, limitless replicative potential, sustained angiogenesis, and tissue invasion and metastasis." They anticipated a future simplification of these "layers of complexity," but subsequent research added more: reprogramming of energy metabolism in the cells and evasion of immune response plus two "enabling traits," genomic instability and mutation (Fouad and Aanei, 2017).

Insightful as this list is, it is still possible to miss obvious factors. Pischinger (1991) pointed out that cutting open the organism to remove a tumor would damage the GRS, leaving a gaping hole. It was for this reason that polysaccharides such as glucosamine sulfate and chondroitin sulfate were introduced in the popular marketplace to strengthen the matrix. Again, lack of perspective leaves out something big and obvious. The former is a by-product of the veal calf industry; the latter is obtained from shark cartilage from the fishing industry. This gave rise to a motto that went around the health food store world in the 1990s: "Sharks don't get cancer." I don't know if this is true, but more importantly, research showed that 70 percent of glucosamine sulfate could get through the small intestine wall, while only 7 percent of chondroitin sulfate made it.

Meanwhile, research was accumulating that showed it was not always necessary for a medicinal agent to even cross the small intestine membrane to have an effect on cancer and other diseases. Thus, for example, the basic components in mushrooms that have a well-documented anticancer activity are the beta glucans, which are polysaccharides from the cell membranes of the fungi. They are not digestible but rub up against the wall of the small intestine, exchanging information with the regulatory system of the cells they are passing by. It may not be the information they exchange, even, that is so curative; it may simply be the method of communication, which reinforces the healthy communication system of the matrix/cell circuitry.

In addition to the cell and the matrix, we also have to include the microbiome of microbes living on the surface on the mucous membranes of the body and also inside the organism. The microbiome also exchanges information with the GRS and the cells of the host organism, for better or worse.

Communication inside the matrix, between the matrix and the cell, and between the matrix and the outside world (the microbiome) are the three main factors contributing to malignancy (Alfano et al. 2016, 77). An even broader survey would place the following causes in the arena:

1. Severe shock of any kind, resulting in the exudation of blood proteins from the vessels into the matrix, overwhelming the immune cells, inviting in bacteria, clogging the matrix, increasing or reducing oxidation, and decreasing communication within the matrix.

2. Poor microcirculation, resulting in weakness of cells and matrix in local areas fed by the capillary bed.

3. Weak immune response, so that damaged and mutated cells are not broken down and removed; poor leukocyte production in the bone marrow, lymphatics, or elsewhere.

4. Prolonged bacterial infections that weaken the immune response, perpetuate the presence of enzymes that break down the matrix, or cause regulatory disruption in the matrix.

5. Prolonged bacterial infections that cause excessive leukocyte production in the bone marrow, resulting in leukemic diseases.

6. Disregulation of the environment of the cells by the GRS, resulting in aberrant cellular behavior. (Here we may see the influence of pharmaceuticals that bypass the GRS to strike directly at the cell membrane.)

7. Damage to the matrix or poor maintenance and remodeling, resulting in contouring that favors cancer cell development, propagation, and movement.

8. Thickening of the matrix environment with collagens, causing congestion, poor elimination, and incorrect signaling.

9. An excessive oxidative environment favoring the breakdown and mutation of cells.

10. A state of low oxidation due to congestion; for example, after a shock or a bruise that leaves dead blood cells in the matrix. Remember that cancer cells do not rely on oxidation but rather fermentation to reproduce.

11. Poor mitochondrial health and performance, so that not enough energy is manufactured to be stored in the cell membrane. Lack of components in the citric acid cycle that generates energy in the mitochondria.

12. Poor encysting of developing cancers by matrix polymers.

13. Excessive growth factors stimulating cancer cell growth.

14. High blood sugar, causing higher levels of IGF-1, or sulfation factor, changing the healthy matrix makeup and providing food for bacteria and mutagenic cells.

15. Toxins coming in from the adjacent microbiome, manufactured by bacterial colonies that are not healthy or normal to the mucous membrane they inhabit.

16. Toxins in the food rubbing up against the cell membranes in the gastrointestinal tract or microbiome to introduce new signaling.
17. Poor elimination through the lymphatic capillaries or venules.

Virtually all of these problems may be positively influenced by keeping the matrix, capillary bed, and lymphatic drainage system strong and healthy. These same problems will also create the myriads of lesser diseases that need attention. We can see, therefore, the ideology of Marguerite Maury and Samuel West, who conceived treatment of all diseases through the matrix, capillaries, and lymphatics. This will be explained in our final chapter, "The In-Mix-Out of the Matrix."

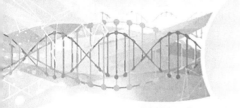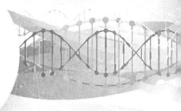

4

The Matrix and Wound Healing
Template for Healing Matrix Injury

Turn your wounds into wisdom.

Oprah Winfrey

Understanding the processes and components involved in the self-healing of wounds and traumas not only facilitates our comprehension of how the matrix builds and repairs itself, but also helps us learn how to treat the ECM in a knowledgeable fashion. A review article titled "The Role of the Extracellular Matrix Components in Cutaneous Wound Healing" (Olczyk, Mencner, and Komosinska-Vassev 2014) gives an excellent overview of the subject. The authors trace out the role of ECM constituents in the progress of wound healing. These constituents play significant roles in hemostasis (stopping bleeding) and each of the three stages of healing: *inflammation, granulation,* and *remodeling.* The whole process includes the building of new "scaffolding," or a "provisional new matrix," various repair processes, with signaling and regulation during this dynamic, interactive sequence. These same processes apply when toxins, microbes, internal wounds, and such attack the matrix—though the bleeding stage will not generally occur.

Many different factors figure into wound healing, including blood platelets and the clotting cascade, immune cells (especially neutrophils and macrophages), fibroblasts and keratinocytes that generate replacement fibers, endothelial cells that rebuild vessel linings, and an array of ECM polymers and fibers. These substances, cells, and activities are regulated by an array of biochemical mediators, including cytokines, leukotrienes, interferons, prostaglandins, growth factors, and other substances that trigger the inflammatory response, cell proliferation, differentiation, growth, and metabolism. The delicate balances in these processes are regulated by stem cells that enhance repair by the secretion of paracrine factors (locally generated hormones at the site of the injury). Stem cells that generate different kinds of cells are also essential.

The "same old characters" we studied before—matrix polymers and fibers—are involved in these activities. Dermatan sulfate enhances the adhesion of leukocytes (white blood cells) in the endothelial level, increases fibroblast and keratinocyte growth factors, and interacts with heparin, platelets, and fibronectin to influence clotting and scab formation. Chondroitin sulfate induces cell proliferation, regulates cell adhesion, and stimulates cell migration. Heparan sulfate/heparin participates in the generation of new blood vessels and the growth, migration, and differentiation of new cells. HA provides the basic new scaffolding for tissue repair, determines local hydration, operates as a GRS signaling medium, interacts with cell membrane receptors, stimulates cell proliferation, migration, and differentiation, and enhances gene expression. As shown in a 2011 article from the *Journal of Wound Care* (see the section "Iodine and Wound Healing" on p. 141), the role of hyaluronins in the healing process demands much more attention.

STOPPING BLEEDING (HEMOSTASIS)

The first step of the healing process is *hemostasis,* or staunching of blood. Ruptured blood vessels activate platelets, beginning a cascade toward the formation of clots that ends in the generation of fibrin and the adhesion of fibrin, cells, and cell parts in the scab. The platelets are activated by contact with the collagen of damaged vessels, and the substances they release include matrix proteins such as fibronectin. The surface of the activated platelets becomes the location for the activation of prothrombin, which begins the cascade—including the transformation of fibrinogen to fibrin—that results in the formation of a blood clot. The clot "protects the structural integrity of vessels and provides a provisional 'scaffolding' which enables formation of a temporary matrix in the wound bed" (Olczyk, Mencner, and Komosinska-Vassev 2014). This new scaffold is composed primarily of hyaluronins, but also fibronectin, which is highly adhesive. The platelets trapped in the provisional matrix release growth factors that recruit neutrophils, macrophages, endothelial cells, and fibroblasts into the area. The neutrophils and macrophages initiate the inflammatory response. Endothelial cells begin the regeneration of capillaries, or angiogenesis. Fibroblasts initiate the migration of these replacement cells into the wound environment, their proliferation, and the manufacture of GAGs and collagen. At the same time, to prevent bleeding, remaining healthy blood vessels are narrowed by vasoconstrictive factors, including serotonin and adrenaline, to prevent blood from flowing into the region.

Hemostatics

The diversity of hemostatic mechanisms explains why there are a variety of herbs suited to different types of wounds. These are called *hemostatics*. In order to use them skillfully, we need to know the differentials in the specific indications. We would use Yarrow (*Achillea millefolium*) when the cut is deep and the wound bleeds freely, Labrador Tea (*Ledum groenlandica*) for puncture wounds with poor aeration and oxidation, Arnica (*Arnica montana*) for a damaged capillary bed resulting in a bruise, Plantain (*Plantago* spp.) as a drawing agent for unclean wounds, St. John's Wort (*Hypericum perforatum*) if nerves are inflamed, injured, and painful, and Red Root (*Ceanothus* spp.) for a wound with seepage. Most of these indications are widely attested.

Salad Burnett (*Sanguisorba officinalis*), Safflower (*Carthamus tinctoria*), and Yarrow appear to exert an influence over the arterioles to direct blood away from the area. They appear to encourage local vasoconstriction, apparently with generalized vasodilation, so that the blood vessels elsewhere can take up the blood and prevent it from gushing from the wound. These indications from my own observations.

We not only want to stop the bleeding, but also begin the building of the new matrix scaffolding. Hemostasis prompts the start of healing.

THE THREE STAGES OF HEALING

Three fundamental stages of healing have long been recognized. They overlap but also follow one another in sequence. The processes associated in a stage can be overactive or underactive, so that the organism gets stuck, and that blocks the later stages from occurring. For instance, no granulation (cell proliferation and regrowth) will occur as long as the area is inflamed. Excessive granulation (commonly called proud flesh) will block the next stage, including the formation of a healthy scar that signals the end of the process.

It will be noticed that many of the most common household herbs are suited to the three stages of healing, including Calendula, Aloe, Echinacea, Propolis, Garlic, Comfrey, Opuntia, Cayenne, and Papaya. However, they are often used in a clumsy manner because their relationships to specific processes in healing have not been explained or absorbed into folk medicine. I have included descriptions of some of these herbs specifically so that they can be used more skillfully.

▸ *The Inflammatory Stage* ◂

Inflammation develops during the first twenty-four hours after an injury has occurred and lasts on average for up to forty-eight hours in a modest wound. The characteristic symptoms of inflammation—established since the doctors of ancient Rome—are redness (*rubor*), heat (*calor*), swelling (*tumor*), and pain (*dolor*). (Sounds better in Latin.)

The inflammatory stage is initiated by neutrophils—the first pro-inflammatory cells to appear at the wound site—and continued by macrophages, the consumers of bacteria and debris. Neutrophils and macrophages are the first line of defense against infections, consuming invading bacteria, the proteases they release, and the debris from injured tissue. They intensify the inflammatory reaction by releasing pro-inflammatory cytokines. They also generate reactive compounds containing oxygen and nitrogen that encourage and control oxidative processes. Thrombin and products of fibrin decomposition, bacteria, cytokines, and leukotrienes control neutrophil and macrophage behaviors. All of these are attracted to the place of damage by various means. Neutrophils and macrophages not only initiate the inflammatory stage but also release cytokines and growth factors that activate fibroblasts and epithelial cells that create conditions for the initiation of the next phase of the healing process: granulation (Olczyk, Mencner, and Komosinska-Vassev 2014).

Bacteria arrive early at the scene as scavengers living off debris. They produce various kinds of proteases (enzymes that break down proteins) in the course of their work. These act on both the matrix itself and the cells. They increase the virulence of infection and the degradation of tissue, and encourage the evasion and destruction of physical barriers to bacterial invasion. Some of them secrete the enzyme hyaluronidase, which breaks down HA, retarding repair and facilitating the spread of bacteria. They also secrete the enzymes collagenase and elastase to break down connective tissue fibers and perpetuate the invasion. These activities spread the bacteria through the matrix, furthering the inflammatory response. Other bacterial enzymes generate free radicals that cause additional inflammation and tissue degradation through uncontrolled oxidation. Neutrophils and macrophages need to contain and remove the bacteria, including their proteases and enzymes, not only to bring the inflammatory stage to an end but also to prevent mutation in the DNA of cells and damage to the matrix, both of which can encourage the eventual appearance of cancer (Alfano et al. 2016).

The blood vessels that had contracted to promote hemostasis are not widened. However, the membranes become more permeable, and plasma diffuses out into the wound to help moisten the incipient matrix scaffold produced by serum-hungry hyaluronins. These changes are supported by histamine, kinins, prostaglandins, leukotrienes, protease enzymes (to break down protein in the scab produced during hemostasis), acid hydrolases, and nitrogen oxide (Olczyk, Mencner, and Komosinska-Vassev 2014).

After a two- or three-day presence in the wound area, the neutrophils are depleted by apoptosis and replaced by monocytes that migrate from the capillaries into matrix. Here they are transformed. The transformative substance for making monocytes into macrophages is thrombin, which is activated in the hemostatic cascade in the blood. Macrophages play a double role in the healing process, participating in phagocytosis and releasing cytokines and growth factors that stimulate the proliferation of fibroblasts and collagens. They also cause the removal of fibrin clots. Moreover, they are the source of mediators that not only control the inflammatory process but also modulate epithelialization, collagen accumulation, and vessel creation. In the late inflammatory phase, lymphocytes also infiltrate the wound environment, influencing fibroblast proliferation and collagen production. An absence of neutrophils and a reduction in the amount of macrophages in the wound indicates that the inflammatory phase is drawing to a close and the proliferation phase is beginning (Olczyk, Mencner, and Komosinska-Vassev 2014).

Remedies that act on the four symptoms of inflammation are well known in herbal medicine. A full range would include those for an overactive immune response as well as those for an underactive response. An incomplete list of remedies for mast cell overreaction is given in chapter 6, while a few for depressed immunity (Calendula, Echinacea) are listed here. Native Americans used and still use saps and resins to seal off, sanitize, and heal wounds. Marguerite Maury (see chapter 6) considered such resins and dense essential oils to be especially active on the matrix. As a class, the herbs used here possess or combine these sedative or stimulating properties with mucilage.

ꝑ *Calendula officinalis* (Calendula)

This plant medicine comes to us from central European folk medicine via homeopathy. It is used in homeopathy in herbal doses, externally, for wound healing. The flowers are used, including the petals (which are slightly sweet and mucilaginous) and the corollas or flower bases (which are bitter and salty).

It is said in many herbal websites and books (I used to say this) that Calendula contains iodine. However, modern assays do not bear this out. What does seem to be true is that Calendula picks up iodine. This is indicated by the fact that it was used, a hundred years ago, to detect the presence of iodine. Calendula tincture turns red in the presence of iodine, according to research by Phyllis Light. This means that there is a chemical reaction between Calendula and iodine. Since there is already iodine in the body, this means that the plant picks up available iodine. This naturally produces the powerful topical or local healing formula discovered by Dr. Keith Cutting and mentioned below that is made of iodine and HA (or mucilage) and is now available as a product called Hyiodine.

Calendula is used for all kinds of surface injuries, cuts, and wounds. It does not have the reputation of Yarrow as a hemostatic. It is best suited to swollen, red, inflamed, painful tissues that are not open, so that pus is building up inside (think of a cat scratch). From experience, we can deduce that Calendula helps with drainage from the wound through the lymphatics. It is an excellent remedy for swollen lymphatics independent of a wound, especially old, stagnant cases needing mild stimulation. But it manifests its herbal genius when there is a surface wound.

Calendula is considered a *bacteriostatic,* meaning that it does not kill bacteria but stabilizes the population of microbes as the wound heals. This means it does not interfere with the natural healing processes associated with natural immunity, which, as we saw above, are very finely tuned by changing sequences of immune cells. The havoc wrecked on the system by antibiotics (more so when taken internally) is impossible to estimate. We know that they destroy the gut flora, leading to almost untreatable conditions like small intestine bacterial overgrowth.

We do not know exactly what Calendula does, but clearly it assists in the removal of pus and the laying down of the new "scaffolding" consisting of matrix polymers analogous to those found in the Calendula petals and also probably has an encouraging or regulatory effect on immune cell activity. At any rate, it is the single most important wound-healing medicine in herbalism.

ॐ *Echinacea* spp.

World-famous Echinacea is a good example of an overused herb, but it has a specific and very well-configured relationship to inflammatory processes. It antidotes hyaluronidase, the enzyme that dissolves HA, while encouraging the growth of HA. This enzyme is released by streptococcus and staphylococcus bacteria. It also is in rattlesnake venom and released by some cancers.

Echinacea possesses a diffusive or tingling taste. Diffusives are stimulants that are not warming (like aromatics with volatile oils), but act more on the nerves. Echinacea's stimulating properties act mostly on the innervation of the veins and lymphatic ducts, which possess a very limited neurological capacity. So it strengthens the matrix and then helps the veins and lymphatics carry away the waste products. It is therefore particularly suited to the prevention or treatment of septic wounds. This is what it was originally used for, not all the theoretical "immune-boosting" properties for which it is advertised today. Yes, it stimulates the immune system, but mostly factors associated with poison and sepsis, not head colds and acute illness.

After they learned about it from the eclectics, German pharmacology set Echinacea on the backburner until the 1980s, when the HIV/AIDS epidemic hit and everybody wanted to "boost their immune system." Echinacea contains immune-boosting substances, but these are suited to septic conditions, not the type of immunity needed to fight off head colds or HIV/AIDS. Therefore, Echinacea has been disappointing in studies trying to demonstrate its usefulness in acute conditions. As a commentator in the *New England Journal of Medicine* complained after a study failed to find positive evidence, the Native Americans and the pioneers did not use it for these acute conditions. This is an important point. Folk medicine should be consulted, along with science.

Speaking of which, Echinacea was used by the Native people and pioneers in feed to strengthen horses. This indicates that it has a nutritive effect as well as being immune boosting.

In addition to its application for infected wounds that are turning septic, Echinacea is also a good external remedy for acute beestings. I think of the bright pink flowers, which have the look of irritated, histaminic skin or mucosa, as a signature here. This suggests that Echinacea is useful for both autoimmune excess and immune deficiency. Many herbs are in fact normalizers between two poles. The antiseptic signature for Echinacea is the black root and the slightly purple color at the end of the flower petals.

Despite Echinacea's popularity, there are still a great many things we need to learn about this amazing plant.

► *The Proliferation or Granulation Stage* ◄

This is the phase in which proliferation of cells occurs so that new connective tissue, epithelium, and endothelial vessel tissue can be laid down. It is also frequently called granulation because the newly laid down capillary bed tufts look like granules. This combination of proliferating cells makes a tissue that is unformed and pink. The work of regrowth and replacement is synergistic as fibroblasts synthesize new ECM components in the presence of newly formed blood vessels manufactured by endothelial cells migrating and proliferating to close up the wound.

Wounds that do not involve the loss of tissue are said to heal by "first intention"—an old Galenic term—and return to a form and condition similar to the original state, while extensive injuries with tissue loss heal by "second intention," forming a scar.

After hemostasis and inflammation, the rebuilding of damaged tissue intensifies. During this stage, the number of cells in the bed of the wound increases due to the migration and proliferation of fibroblasts, endothelial cells, and keratinocytes, all of which secrete growth factors.

These mediators stimulate and modulate the rebuilding of the matrix, the generation of new blood vessels, and their covering by epithelial cells.

Granulation is divided into three distinct activities. During (1) matrix biosynthesis, the scaffolding of the matrix is rebuilt. This is followed by (2) epithelialization, when a covering membrane is reestablished. This needs to be supported by new blood vessels so it is supplemented by (3) angiogenesis. These activities are complex, but they are important to understand, since there are herbs that are fairly specific to all three. I have relied upon Olczyk, Mencner, and Komosinska-Vassev (2014) for the following presentation.

Step 1 of Granulation: Matrix Biosynthesis

In this first stage, a temporary matrix is formed, mainly by fibrin and fibronectins; later, it is replaced by collagen matrix and enriched with PGs, GAGs, and noncollagenous glycoproteins. This allows the restoration of structure and function in the regrowing tissue.

The key cells in the granulation phase are the fibroblasts. They are formed mainly from undifferentiated cells residing in the skin. Under the influence of cytokines and growth factors released from blood platelets, neutrophils, and macrophages, these undifferentiated cells undergo a transformation into fibroblasts. In the forty-eight to seventy-two hours after an injury, these cells migrate to the site of the trauma, attracted by growth factors (PDGF, EGF, IGF-1, and TGF-β) that also stimulate the proliferation of these cells. With their arrival, the synthesis of matrix components and the formation of granulation starts. Granulated tissue appears about the fourth day after the injury.

The collagen, elastin, PGs, GAGs, and noncollagenous proteins are mainly synthesized by the fibroblasts, whose activity is regulated by PDGF and TGF-β growth factors. PDGF originates mainly from blood platelets and macrophages. It also stimulates the work of collagenase, an enzyme that breaks down collagen, while TGF-β, also secreted by blood platelets and macrophages, regulates the accumulation of matrix components at the site of injury.

The matrix of early granulation tissue (up to the third day after the injury) contains a large amount of HA and fibronectin. The former creates a woven structure that enables the arriving cells to penetrate the wound area. The fibronectin creates scaffolding that facilitates the genesis of collagen. Starting with the third day after the injury, the concentration of HA within the wound area quickly decreases, and collagen fibers take over. The amount of collagen in the granulation tissue increases up to the third week from the time of the wound and is accompanied by a gradual decrease of the number of fibroblasts, up to the moment when they disappear in the process of apoptosis.

The dominant kinds of collagen in the skin are types I and III. They occur in a proportion of 4:1, but during the initial phases of healing, type III predominates. This collagen "toughens" the newly created tissue, giving it tensile strength. The granulating tissue is also enriched by the presence of heparan sulfate proteoglycans, which appear in the wound area a few hours after the injury. PGs chondroitin sulfate and dermatan sulfate appear in the wound area significantly later, in the second week of the healing process. The granulation tissue, temporarily substituting for the dermis, ultimately matures into a scar during the remodeling phase. It has a thick network of vessels and capillaries and a significant amount of cells, including macrophages and fibroblasts as well as collagen fibers. These are arranged without order in the wound. Granulation tissue is characterized by a faster metabolism, compared with the dermis, because of all the cell migration, replication, and intensified protein synthesis (Olczyk, Mencner, and Komosinska-Vassev 2014).

A number of problems can occur due to difficulties in granulation. An excess of granulation can form. This is called proud flesh in folk medicine: it usually occurs due to dirty wounds, so it is much more common today in animals than people. Occasionally, it occurs as a side effect of surgery; this is the only way I have seen it brought on in the modern human population. Another problem occurs when the wound is too wet, releasing ECFs constantly so that granulation cannot occur. I have used Elecampane (*Inula helenium*) for proud flesh.

Herbs to Support Matrix Biosynthesis

ࣹ Aloe vera

This succulent has been used in medicine since ancient times. The layer under the external rind contains a yellow substance rich in anthroquinones, so that it is cathartic, while the inner gel contains 99 percent water mixed with glucomannans (akin to matrix polysaccharides), amino acids, lipids, sterols, electrolytes, and vitamins. The gel has been used in folk medicine as a wound medicine and burn remedy. It is excellent for burns when used in a spray freshly prepared from the gel and water, notes herbalist Steven Horne.

The name *Aloe* derives from the Arabic *alloeh,* meaning "shining bitter substance," while the word *vera* means "true" in Latin. The Egyptians called Aloe the "plant of immortality," and the Greeks regarded it as a universal panacea. It is also used in traditional medicine in China, India, and Mexico. It is a member of the Asphodel family in the greater Lily clan. A review article in the *Indian Journal of Dermatology,* drawing on several studies, characterized the mechanism of action of the healing properties of Aloe as follows:

> Glucomannan, a mannose-rich polysaccharide, and gibberellin, a growth hormone, interacts with growth factor receptors on the fibroblast, thereby stimulating its activity and proliferation, which in turn significantly increases collagen synthesis after topical and oral Aloe vera. Aloe gel not only increased collagen content of the wound but also changed collagen composition (more type III) and increased the degree of collagen cross linking. Due to this, it accelerated wound contraction and increased the breaking strength of resulting scar tissue. An increased synthesis of hyaluronic acid and dermatan sulfate in the granulation tissue of a healing wound

following oral or topical treatment has been reported. (Surjushe, Vasani, and Saple 2008, 163–66)

In addition, it contains many other anti-inflammatory components and the growth stimulant gibberellin. Natural gibberellins, from willow branches, are used in the nursery industry to root branches to grow into trees. The polysaccharides help moisten the skin and Aloe is believed to have a protective influence against UV and gamma radiation.

In a study published in *Wounds,* it was shown that *Aloe vera* in vitro "had significant stimulatory effects on cell proliferation and migration of both fibroblasts and keratinocytes." Unexpectedly, it also showed "strong protective effects" on keratinocytes that had been exposed to toxins. "The results suggest *A. vera* accelerates wound healing by promoting proliferation and migration of fibroblasts and keratinocytes and by protecting keratinocytes" (Teplicki et al. 2018).

ࣺ *Centella asiatica* (Gotu Kola)

Gotu Kola is now one of the most widely used and trusted herbs in popular medicine, but I still remember when it was introduced in the 1990s. It is a tonic that is safe and easy to use. It can be used as a general, nonspecific tonic for health, especially of the brain. It is a geriatric herb in India and China, where it is well known.

In addition to a long history of use, Gotu Kola also sports a sizable record of research. A good review article was published by the *Indian Journal of Pharmaceutical Sciences* (Gohil, Patel, and Gajjar 2010).

The saponins or triterpenoids, including asiaticosides, are widely considered to be the major active ingredients in Gotu Kola. They are believed to be responsible for the wound healing and vascular effects for which the plant is known first and foremost and to work by inhibiting the production of collagen at the wound site. In addition, *Centella* contains sterols, flavonoids, tannins, mucilages, free amino acids, glutamate, lysine, an alkaloid, a bitter, and essential fatty acids.

Although it is a general tonic, Gotu Kola possesses some specific properties and organ affinities and has an energetic profile (cooling and drying). It eliminates excess fluids, shrinks swollen tissues, neutralizes acids in the fluids, lowers body temperature, improves the health of blood vessels, and decreases fatigue, depression, and anxiety. It has more of an affinity to the CNS than the ANS. By simultaneously cooling inflammation and repairing tissue, it is widely useful, certainly in wounds. It acts on inflammation and then the first and second stages of wound healing that follow (rebuilding the scaffold, keratinization), so it is no wonder it reduces scar tissue (the third stage). Furthermore, it acts on the matrix polymers—the GAGs in particular—so that it can further rebuilding and wound repair and tighten and tone tissues.

Gotu Kola contains flavonoids that reduce the heat and inflammation caused by excess oxidation, while at the same time, from the presence of asiaticoside, it keeps the blood vessels healthy (they tend to get beat up in inflammatory conditions) and repairs connective tissue, matrix polymers, fibers, ligaments, cartilage, bones, arteries, and veins. It is, as a consequence, recommended in cardiovascular and circulatory disorders, varicosities, liver problems (an organ that needs constant cooling and rebuilding and relies on an extensive venous network), and kidney stones (an organ needing an extensive arterial/capillary network). It has been used to treat phlebitis (inflammation of the veins), leg cramps, swelling of the legs, and heaviness or tingling in the legs.

Gotu Kola acts on the most ancient and primal tissues of the body, the polymers of the matrix that bind together the cells and regulate cellular activity, so it is deeply active, as its reputation suggests. It also acts on connective tissues. When these tissues become sclerotic, they produce arthritic and muscular pain, including fibromyalgia, for which Gotu Kola is a general, nonspecific tonic remedy. This means it would also improve the piezoelectric communication system (the biomechanical regulatory system) operating through connective tissue.

Among the connective tissues it acts on, Gotu Kola has a strong affinity for the skin; it has been found effective in skin problems from mild inflammation to leprosy. *Centella* is used topically for wound healing, burns, and the stimulation of hair and nail growth, and it is supportive in the repair of cartilage. The asiaticoside in it helps dissolve the protective coating around the leprosy bacteria so that the immune system can destroy them. It reduces cellulite by increasing the strength of the matrix polymers. It helps in the recovery of skin grafts and is reparative in episiotomy. It can relieve the red welts of psoriasis.

Gotu Kola is widely classified as a nerve tonic. Since it acts so strongly on the connective tissue system, it is tempting to suggest that it acts on the myelin sheaths of the nerve cells or even on the glioblasts, which are modified fibroblasts that generate nerve tissue. Because it is relaxing and improves memory and has improved people's tests scores in studies, Gotu Kola is considered suitable for treatment of ADD. It is also often used for recovery after mental breakdowns, and used regularly, it may prevent nervous breakdowns in the first place. It is calmative in cases of insomnia.

Gotu Kola grows in ditches in India and elsewhere where toxins are prevalent, so it should be obtained from plants grown commercially in Hawaii. Recently, it was discovered that a Gotu Kola native to Mississippi, *Centella erecta,* is as high or higher in active ingredients than the commonly used species. This information comes from herbalist Darryl Martin, who sells it through Blue Boy Herbs.

☙ *Opuntia* spp. (Prickly Pear)

This is not an herb I had experience with when I began my studies of the matrix—it is barely found in Minnesota—but I quickly realized I had overlooked a valuable herb that was ideally suited for use in increasing the health of the matrix.

Not having the benefit of an extensive background in *Opuntia,* I first turned to Michael Moore's *Medicinal Plants of the Desert and Canyon West* (1989, 89). His uses derive directly from Mexican and New Mexican folk medicine and are therefore based on experience.

To this, he added his own extensive experience. The most simple and characteristic use is made of the mucilage in the slimy pads. For a scientifically comprehensive account, I turned to the article "Food as Medicine; Prickly Pear Cactus (Opuntia ficus-indica, Cactaceae)" (Bauman and Schmidt 2015) in *HerbalGram* magazine. This article is not based on experience, but merely on research. The authors completely omit the presence or use of the mucilage from the discussion in their article. This shows the difference between herbal medicine, which values simple substances such as tannins and mucilage, and pharmacology, which does not.

Moore, a practicing herbalist, speaks of the application of the plant in the present tense, which is correct: it is widely used in Latin communities in Mexico and the southwestern United States. Bauman and Schmidt follow the vocabulary of science, which speaks of the herbal and folk uses in the past tense. This is not only disempowering but also actually lacks scientific accuracy since the pads are found in almost all Latin grocery stores. I have seen the pink flower buds, which are stronger antidiabetics, for sale at $85 a gallon in high-end Anglo stores, as well.

I don't mean to pick on Bauman and Schmidt—their article was very useful—but they demonstrate the disconnect between practitioners with experience and scholars without. Regular medicine doesn't think about mucilage, so it "doesn't exist." In this section, I will rely on Moore's account and the use of the mucilage in the pads, while in the section on the mast cells we will discuss the anti-inflammatory and antidiabetic uses mentioned by Bauman and Schmidt.

Opuntia spp. are native to Mexico and much of the United States. I have seen the herb on the hills above Duluth, Minnesota, where it is cold, cold, cold in the winter and cool, cool, cool in the summer. It is naturalized in Australia and South Africa. It is raised as a food and medicinal crop in Mexico.

The flower, fruit, and pad of Opuntia are all used. All have thorns or hairs that have to be removed. The Cactaceae evolved from the

Rosaceae, so it is not surprising to see the same cooling, antifebrile properties in Prickly Pear that we find in the Rose clan. The pads and the fruits both contain a slimy mucilage; the fruits and flower possess the flavonoids.

The fruits and pads have a known antiviral and immune modulating or enhancing effect. Studies have shown improvement in platelet function. The pads are less high in flavonoids, but they are certainly cooling and anti-inflammatory. Both the fruits and the pads are slimy, showing the presence of mucilaginous polysaccharides. The pads contain manganese, which is essential in glucose metabolism, as well as the antispasmodic magnesium, vitamin C, and the massive amounts of mucilage for which they are so well known.

The pads are "filleted," as Moore says, to be used topically on burns and wounds, but are also widely eaten as a food in Mexico and the southwestern United States. The pads cool and lubricate the digestive tract, increasing fluid removal (like Glauber's salts). Anyone can determine this for themselves by picking or buying and eating Opuntia.

Like many wet/salty plants, Opuntia is a cooling diuretic that acts on both the kidneys and the bladder. It is traditionally used for edema and to help stones pass, so it vies with Marshmallow Root for the title "most mucilaginous diuretic" or "most diuretic mucilage." Moore gives a specific indication in cystitis: pain lingering after urination. It is used as a cooling expectorant in bronchitis and asthma, soothing excess coughing or bringing up dried mucus. The pads (or extract) moisten the skin and are a diaphoretic cooling remedy in fever. They have traditionally been used for hangover, which suggests that the pads accelerate catabolic activity, but they are also used for anemia and nutrition, so they have the matching anabolic property as well. The pads have a reputation in vitiligo (localized loss of pigmentation in the skin), abdominal fluid accumulation, tumors, anemia, ulcers, hemorrhoids, prostate enlargement, inflammation of the eyes, lower back pain, and enlargement of the spleen (Bauman and Schmidt 2015).

I don't have any experience with Opuntia, but here is a case history related to me by a friend. Leta Worthington, who ran an herb shop in Austin years ago, told me about a tall young man (the sulfation factor build) with HIV who stuck the pads on his head and got great regrowth of hair. This was, unfortunately, in the days before effective HIV treatment, and he died with a great head of hair. I don't mean to make light of such a sad story, but it is the kind of case history that is memorable.

๛ Carica papaya (Papaya)

This tropical plant is a well-known folk remedy. I have not used it, so I will fall back on the testimony of the late, great Australian herbalist Dorothy Hall, with whom I concur in so many matters medicinal. Dorothy particularly recommended the use of a Papaya ointment. Papaya—they call it "Pawpaw" down there—adjusts the amount of water in the wound up or down, so that it is indicated in wounds that are too moist or too dry. In either case, the healing process is stopped by wrong conditions in the environment. Control of water in the matrix depends on HA and sodium salts. In addition, Papaya contains a vast amount of enzymes that can catalyze activities in the wound. Dorothy raved about the effectiveness in Papaya in many wounds and conditions of the skin.

I used to be a canoe guide, and one of the things I remember about wounds is that when they get wet, they get inflamed and stay infected for a longer time. We can equally imagine that dry matrix polymers are not going to heal quickly either. This may be more of a problem in Australia, where Dorothy practiced.

๛ Propolis (Bee Secretion)

This natural product of the beehive is made from resins collected by bees from tree buds, especially in the Poplar branch of the Willow family. The bees return to the hive, vomit up the digested, remade resin, and use it to patch holes in the hive. Its powerful antimicrobial properties make it perfect for protection and regrowth of superficial tissue. As a resin, Propolis fits the profile of the agents (resins and heavy volatile oils) that act strongly on the matrix, according to Marguerite Maury and Native American wound healing traditions. It seems to have enjoyed its most popularity as a medicinal herb (if we think of it as tree resins) in Eastern Europe and the Middle East.

The analogy of bee usage to human application is so obvious that it hardly needs science to tell us to use Propolis to repair surfaces and rid membranes of various invasive critters. Indeed, Propolis has been used as medicine since the Bronze Age. At one archaeological site, it was found combined with seeds of *Nigella sativa,* which would make a truly formidable healing agent indeed (Salih, Sipahi, and Dönmez 2009).

Propolis has been studied a great deal in modern research, although it suffers from a problem that does not suit it well to the modern model: no two batches of Propolis are identical, since they are made from bees collecting resins in different areas and times.

Research has shown, however, that Propolis acts particularly strongly on fibronectins and collagens I and III, which are very important in this stage of wound healing. At the end of their article, Olczyk, Mencner, and Komosinska-Vassev (2014) mention research they have undertaken using Propolis to hasten and improve wound healing. They say that it "accelerates the burned tissue repair by stimulation of the wound bed GAG accumulation needed for granulation, tissue growth, and wound closure." In addition, it "accelerates chondroitin/dermatan sulfates" that encourage the "structure modification responsible for binding growth factors playing a crucial role in the tissue repair." The authors maintain that matrix constituents, such as collagen, GAGs, fibronectin, and laminin, produce better healing effects when natural therapeutic agents such as Propolis are used, rather than silver sulfadiazine, the "so-called 'gold standard' in topical wound management."

Propolis is widely used for diseases of the surface: oral health (disinfectant mouthwash), laryngitis (an excellent voice restorer), respiratory infection (I would associate it with "hot, raw bronchitis"), mucosal health in the gastrointestinal tract, vaginal health, including recurrent candida, and skin care. It is particularly active in fibronectin processes supporting healthy growth and wound healing.

Propolis resembles a complete apothecary. It is composed of resin (50 percent), wax (30 percent), essential oils (10 percent), pollen (5 percent), and other organic compounds (5 percent). The last category includes phenolic compounds (caffeic acid and cinnamic acid), esters, flavonoids, terpenes, beta-steroids, aromatic aldehydes, and alcohols. It contains no less than twelve flavonoids, including many common to plants: rutin, quercetin, acacetin, chrysin, luteolin, kaempferol, apigenin, myricetin, catechin, and galangin. It also contains vitamins B1, B2, B6, C, and E, and minerals such as magnesium, calcium, potassium, sodium, copper, zinc, manganese, and iron. It also contains resveratrol.

Step 2 of Granulation: Epithelialization

Epithelial cells proliferate above the basement membrane to produce skin and mucosa. They participate in closing the wound surface and growing tissue outward from both the wound edges and epithelial appendages (such as hair follicles, sweat glands, or sebaceous glands) to reconstruct the epithelium after the injury. Some epithelial cells detach themselves from their original places, migrate to the wound area, proliferate, and differentiate. Only cells lying directly on a basement membrane are able to proliferate in this way. They also "deliver" new cells to the new epithelial layer above, as it is being created. Cell migration lasts up to the moment when the epithelial cells are all connected together to create a uniform layer. The mediators that stimulate migration and proliferation are growth factors (EGF, KGF, TGF-α, etc.). The growth factor that accelerates the "maturation" of the epithelial cell layers is TGF-β.

In addition to epithelial cells, keratinocytes are involved in the reconstruction of healthy epithelium. They separate from the basement membrane and migrate up into the higher layers. Various enzymes degrade the collagen type IV of the basement membrane and the collagen type VII that creates anchoring fibrils in the membrane.

Herb to Support Epithelialization

৯ *Symphytum officinale* (Comfrey)

The ability of Comfrey to repair damaged surfaces is so famous that it hardly needs comment; it probably has more affinity to the process of epithelialization than any other known plant medicine. It will even cause calluses to grow on skin overnight, thickening the layers above the basement membrane. It also is famous for the treatment of ulceration of the mucosa and probably acts on other mucosal difficulties where the epithelium needs stimulation. A similar effect occurs on serous and synovial membranes, which are also epithelial. As we have seen, these form boundaries in and around the matrix, organs, and tissues. The constituent which is responsible for this rapid growth is allantoin, which has been shown to have the ability to proliferate both epithelium and keratocytes, so it is exactly suited to this phase of granulation. Borage, a cousin of Comfrey, possesses this allantoin-based super-power as well. Solomon's Seal also contains allantoin.

In addition to stimulating growth via allantoin, Comfrey is rich is tannins, so it is an astringent. This has a secondary curative action, drawing substances to the area of repair. In cartilaginous material, which has no direct blood supply in or out, Comfrey draws the fluids through the joints, increasing nutrition and elimination. This is very important. Because these tissues don't have a circulatory system, they have to rely on the same gentle movements that stir the waters of the matrix.

Because Comfrey does not stimulate circulation of the blood, it can cause overgrowth and even necrosis of the tissues if the following step is lagging behind. This is why it is traditional to give Comfrey for ulcers with a small amount of Cayenne (*Capsicum annuum*).

Step 3 of Granulation: Angiogenesis

The creation of new blood vessels is called *angiogenesis*. These new vessels restore blood circulation to the area of damage, bringing in oxygen, food supplies, and reparative cells, preventing the development of necrosis and tissue death from lack of oxygen. When cancer is present, we often try to slow angiogenesis to prevent its spread, but most of the time we want to promote angiogenesis to encourage the growth and repair of healthy tissues.

Angiogenesis is stimulated by low oxygen levels, low pH levels (tissue acidity), or high lactic acid concentration. In addition, mediators soluble in the ECFs—bFGF, TGF-β, TNF-α, VEGF, angiogenin, and angiotropin secreted by epithelial cells, fibroblasts, endothelial cells, and macrophages—produce a strong proangiogenic activity.

The regulation of angiogenesis includes both growth factors and inhibition factors. The latter include angiostatin and thrombospondin. HA molecules of low molecular mass induce angiogenesis, while those of a big molecular mass exert the activity in the opposite direction.

Angiogenesis constitutes a key step in the process of healing. It is not completely separate from the other steps in the healing process. As different groups of endothelial cells conjoin together, they create a structure that provides the beginning for a new blood vessel loop. This process continues until the capillary bed has been restored and the correct amount of oxygen is again flowing into the tissues, along with the nutrients needed to maintain the restored wound environment. Visible capillary tufts give the wound surface the granular appearance that is the origin of the term *granulation*. When the tissue is replaced by a new collagen matrix and, in the last phase, by a scar, requirements for oxygen and nutrients are significantly lower, so there is a lessening need for capillaries. Angiogenesis stops and a part of the capillary bed disintegrates through apoptosis. This is a sluggish process, so reduction of the color of the scar can take many years. If there is an herb that is suited to reducing this effect, I do not know its name. However, remedies that increase angiogenesis include *Lavandula* spp. (Lavender), *Capsicum annuum* (Cayenne), and *Sassafras albidum* (Sassafras).

Herb to Support Angiogenesis

?❧ *Lavandula* spp. (Lavender)

The Lavender clan is a unique and useful subdivision of the mint family. There are not many mints that are as strongly cooling as the Lavenders; in addition, they are sedative. They are some of the few medicinal plants that have almost always been used as oils rather than in typical herbal teas or tinctures. The oil has a beautiful scent, but the flowers and leaves have a bitter taste, so they don't make a pleasant beverage. The bitter flavor allows us to classify this plant as a "cooling bitter," like Yarrow or Goldenseal.

Several Lavenders are native to the Mediterranean region, but they are cultivated in many other places. They can overwinter even in Minnesota, but they do not flourish like they would elsewhere. They are small woody plants or shrubs, with a cluster of woody, perennial stems, like Rosemary. The oil is developed in the leaves and moved to the flowers for storage; it contains linalyl acetate (30–50 percent), linalool, borneol (small amounts), isoborneol, cineole, and camphor. The overall smell is clean, and the name comes from *lavan,* "to clean." The great Gascon herbalist Maurice Messegue recounted how his mother threw the dried flower tops between sheets and clothes that were being stored to keep them smelling fresh.

Our old friend, the doctrine of signatures, does make merry with this plant. The heads look a little like snakes' heads, giving rise to the name Asp Lavender, and *Lavandula* has been used as a snakebite antidote. Messegue remembered that the hunting dogs, coming home with snakebites, were treated with Lavender oil; but the European snakes don't hold a candle to our North American copperheads, rattlers, and diverse other deadly serpents, so I wouldn't rely on Lavender in this regard.

Dietrich Gümbel (1993, 213) has, I believe, the best and most remarkable explanation for the properties of this plant: "the oil causes an extension of blood vessels," especially the capillaries and veins. This is a remarkable and different way to cool, since an expanded capillary bed and the increased ability to carry the blood away through an expanded venous system automatically cools the peripheral circulation in a fashion unlike any other agent I have ever heard about. The capillary bed is dynamic and ever changing. If we gain a pound of flesh, we gain a million miles of capillaries; if we lose a pound, we lose a million. But this is not all. By increasing the capillary bed, more blood is brought into an area and made available to the tissues so that, as Gümbel says, Lavender has a "connective effect between blood and tissue." Bringing more blood, insulin, and blood sugar past more cells in the periphery means that Lavender will have a hypoglycemic effect—lowering glucose in the blood. In the liver, however, it means there will be more clean, good arterial blood, along with the removal of processed venous blood, so that liver function is intensified. This includes anabolism and catabolism, building and eliminating, so that the liver and the peripheral circulation cool, nourish, and cleanse the tissues. Also, the production of bile is increased, and this promotes digestion of fats and oils.

Gümbel also identifies a heightened effect on the mind. The thin-walled venule (the tail end of the capillary), in the choroid process, is where blood is seeped into the ventricles to become the CSF that coats, soothes, and keeps clean the nerves in the myelin sheaths. These fed the CNS directly with the sugar, oxygen, and electrolytes necessary to maintain good electrical transmission along the neurons. One does, in fact, feel a heightening, refreshing feeling in the mind from the use of Lavender oil, but one also feels cooling and sedative effects because of the increase in the peripheral circulation (bringing blood to the surface to discharge heat), so that the oil applied externally is an excellent remedy for insomnia and mental overactivity. "It is a classical harmonizing, regenerating sedative for the nerves" (Gümbel 1993, 214).

▸ *The Remodeling Stage* ◂

This is the last phase of the healing process, during which the wound surface is contracted. In this stage, the granulated tissue is modified from a loose, weak tissue into a strong, contracted scar. The number of capillaries is reduced as they aggregate into larger vessels. The amount of GAGs and PGs diminishes, as does the water content that fluffed them up. Cell density and metabolic activity are lowered. The proportion of collagen types changes, the total collagen content increases, the spatial organization becomes arranged, and the cross-linkage increases, producing tensile strength in the tissue.

The key factor in the formation of the contracture is the transformation of preexisting fibroblasts into myofibroblasts that produce smooth muscle actin microfilaments that (like muscles) cause cellular contraction. During the second week of normal healing, myofibroblasts become the most numerous cell types in the granulation mass. There is a slow evolution, over several months, from a coarse to a more refined scar, so that the matrix that forms resembles a mature dermis. Macrophages and neutrophils consume broken-down material during this process. These and other cells active in these processes are regulated by cytokines, growth factors, and matrix constituents.

ࣔ Dipsacus sylvestris, D. fullonum (Teasel)

In my experience, Teasel (*Dipsacus fullonum*), White Oak bark (*Quercus alba*), and Wormwood (*Artemisia absinthium*) are beneficial in "neatening up" scar tissue. Wild Bergamot or Sweet Leaf (*Monarda fistulosa*) was taught to us in Minnesota by Tis Mal Crow, a Muskogee medicine man, as the great remedy for preventing and reducing scar tissue from burns. As a burn remedy, Lavender oil and *Monarda* are a good combination.

I have seen Teasel reduce a large scar to half its size. This is a remarkable remedy because it helps the body "remember the blueprint of health." I offer this simply as an observation that people can work with or ignore. I plan to write about this in the future. In addition, we now know that Teasel expels foreign objects from the body, even large ones. This is probably how it happens to reduce scar tissue, some of which, laid down in the remodeling phase, is redundant or excessive.

An interesting thing about Teasel that I did not know until recently—when case histories were sent to me by other herbalists—is that it is a "drawing agent" that will pull substances like glass, metal, and large splinters from the tissues while controlling inflammation. In this respect, it is similar to Plantain, an astringent mucilage.

IODINE IN WOUND HEALING

Iodine has long been used in folk and professional medicine as an antiseptic on wounds, but recent research shows that it also interacts in important ways with hyaluronic acid to facilitate matrix health and healing. An article on wound healing and the matrix published in the *Journal of Wound Cure* by Dr. Keith Cutting (2011, and no, I did not make that name up) showed the importance of a single element, iodine, in the repair of the matrix from trauma.

Some attempt had been made to harness the natural healing ability of HA, but this had not proved effective until iodine was added. The combination turned out to be serendipitous. It resulted in the creation of a new topical healing product called Hyiodine. This substance—I hesitate to call it a "drug" because it is so natural—is a viscous gel composed of HA (in the form of sodium hyaluronate), atomic iodine, and potassium iodide. The hyaluronans and iodine are not chemically bonded but merely delivered in close association with each other.

I am not in the habit of quoting drug advertising materials, but the advertising for Hyiodine is quite educational. The company's website (hyiodine.hu) states that Hyiodine is "based on scientific knowledge of the natural process of tissue repair" and gives the following explanation for the operation of the product:

> As hyaluronic acid has the ability to bind large amounts of fluid, it also plays an important role in the wound healing process. After application of Hyiodine to the wound, the hyaluronic acid draws fluid from the wound (called exudate) and, with it, also draws

growth and nutritional factors from the healthy area around the wound, which are substances positively affecting the healing process. This process results in the concentration of these essential substances in the wound, which improves the healing process. The naturally moist environment created by hyaluronic acid in the wound also promotes cell renewal and growth. (Hyiodine 2019, 2021)

One of the standard medical uses of potassium iodide is in a syrup to thin the mucus in bronchitis, making it less adhesive and easier to expectorate. Mucin is a secretion of the matrix containing a lot of hyaluronins, so we see how, analogously, the iodine is working to facilitate the moist flowability of HA in the Hyiodine. At the same time, it "helps to stabilize hyaluronic acid in the product and prevents its degradation by bacteria" (Hyiodine 2019, 2021). Does it do this for the matrix as well as the product? This suggests that the presence of iodine is of even greater importance than we might otherwise think. Iodine's reputation as an antioxidant, antiseptic, and antimicrobial is well established.

The sodium in Hyiodine also has a purpose. Sodium draws water to itself and therefore draws water into the HA it is compounded with in this product. The emollients or softening remedies in herbal medicine are all salty mucilages that combine sodium with matrix polymers and fibers.

The combination of iodine, sodium, and HA occurs naturally and readily in Nature. Sea vegetables contain high levels of polysaccharide polymers, iodine, and sodium and have long been used for profound healing, not only of wounds but also of deteriorated matrix materials in joints, tendons, bones, and tissues in general.

In addition to these wonderful properties, iodine helps ensure the proper apoptosis of the old, worn-out cell. It has been shown to help remove even malignant and diseased cells that, otherwise, were not getting the apoptotic nudge. This function, however, occurs through the production of thyroid hormone and the proper regulation of cells through hormone messaging. There may be similar messages that help breakdown old matrix polymers. Iodine brings life through warmth and circulation and then ends it through cleansing and apoptosis.

The remedies here include the great family of seaweeds, which contain vast amounts of mucilage and iodine, compared with all our other herbs. Applying seaweed extract to wounds and worn-out tissue has proved highly regenerative. Excellent, readable articles, based on personal experience, are given by Dr. Ryan Drum, an herbalist living surrounded by seaweed on Washington State's Waldron Island, at his website: ryandrum.com.

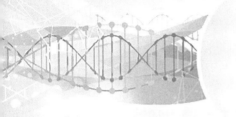
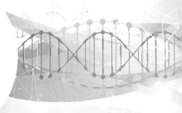

5

Inhabitants of the Matrix

Cells, Tissues, and Organs

*The concept of a cell is, strictly speaking, only a morpho-
logical abstraction. Seen from a biological viewpoint, a cell
cannot be considered by itself without taking its environment into account.*

ALFRED PISCHINGER (2009, 3)

The cell is surrounded by the glycocalyx, which is directly connected to
the matrix polymers, which are made from the same kind of material
and also negatively charged. The glycocalyx receives signals in the form
of electric potential changes that communicate with the lipid-protein
membrane of the cell to open and close receptor sites. The cell membrane is positively charged on the outside and negatively charged on the
inside. It maintains a resting charge that alters with the signal, which
then travels on through the membrane, into the cell, and then to the
cytoskeleton. The latter is composed of the same sort of polymers found
in the matrix and the glycocalyx. The signals are finally conveyed to
the proteins of the cell that hold the codes for different physiological
reactions.

The nucleus stores the genetic codes for cell replication in the
DNA molecules and the codes for life maintenance and survival activities in the RNA molecules. If the matrix signal tells the cell to repro-

duce, the DNA molecules react and begin their subdivision. Most of the time, however, the signal from the matrix interacts with the RNA molecules for the purpose of maintaining ongoing life processes in the cell. The RNA sends signals in the form of messenger proteins (mRNA) that cross back out of the nucleus to the rough endoplasmic reticulum, which surrounds it. Then the mRNA adheres to a ribosome and the instructions are translated into amino acid proteins on the ribosome that travel forth in vacuoles ("little bubbles") through the cytoplasm (internal fluid) of the cell to an organelle ("little organ") called the Golgi apparatus. There, enzymes make protein chains that are destined to remain within the cell to perform cellular functions or are taken to the cell membrane (in vacuoles) for export to the outside of the cell. Some of them attach to the glycocalyx, while others extrude out into the ECM to become the polymers of the matrix.

The mRNA messenger proteins moved from scientific footnote to front page notoriety in 2020, when they were used (instead of viral proteins) to make the coronavirus vaccines. The mRNA proteins selected mimicked those that the virus used to bind to the mucous membrane, to enter the body.

Under a signal from the matrix, via the glycocalyx, glucose is taken up by receptors on the cell membrane. This is the food or fuel of cell life. It is sent to the mitochondria, little bodies that process blood sugar to produce energy with the assistance of oxygen. The combination of fuel plus oxygen plus enzymes continues the ongoing generation of energy, which is stored in chemical bonds (in the ADP/ATP cycle)* and transferred to the cell membrane for storage.

In addition to all its other functions, the cell membrane is a "battery" for the storage of energy. Like any battery, it has a positive and negative pole. The outside is positive, the inside negative. Energy is stored in a polarized form so that excess electrons can flow from the positive pole while the negative will take up energy. This is the basis

---

*ADP is adenosine diphosphate; ATP is adenosine triphosphate.

of energy storage in the cell. Changes in the electrical potential in the matrix, along with sunlight interacting with the structured water that is the main component of the membrane, also change the charge on these cell membranes (Overton 2018).

Electrons do not require channels or pumps because the polymers are semiconductors along which the electrons move, but other substances that enter the cell need special passageways. The usual explanation for their entry involves "pumps" and "channels," but the new research by Gerald Pollack (see chapter 2) suggests that these substances are interactive with the gel-like structured water of the cell membrane and the cytoplasm.

Glucose is water soluble, but there are also fats, oils, and fat-soluble hormones that need to get into the cell. They enter through different receptor sites on the cell membrane, then make their way to another organelle, the smooth endoplasmic reticulum. Both water- and fat-soluble substances travel through the cell plasma in vacuoles.

The gel-like cytoplasm is full of microtubules that resemble the matrix polymers; they are called the cytoskeleton. This forms a complex with the cell plasma, much like how the plasma in the matrix is complexed with matrix polymers. The intracellular plasma is patrolled by lysosomes, or "cleaning bodies" (*lysis,* "cleaning," *soma,* "body"), that clean the interior of the cell.

Many of the processes we have just described require the magical little porphyrins we mentioned previously, which are essential for all oxygen and electric events occurring in the biological sphere. This includes changes in the electrical potential used to signal the exchange of oxygen at the cell membrane and in the mitochondria, as well as the storage of electric charges in the cell membranes.

CELLULAR ANATOMY

Most modern textbooks on cell biology represent the cell as a bag of salty water with little organs (organelles) floating around, enclosed in a skin-like membrane (Overton 2018). The work of Gerald Pollack (2001) challenges this perspective; we now know that the "bag" is filled with structured gel and polymers, as well as the organelles, and is semipermeable with the surrounding matrix. This is a new way to think of the cell, and I will try to describe it from this perspective. However, in reading and rereading my writing, I continually see how much I am bound in the old conception, which separated the cell and the matrix more rigidly than seems to be the reality of the situation.

Cell Membrane: The first thing we need to know about the membrane is that it is not a skin-like boundary, but more like a saturated sponge that interacts with the gel/polymer environments on both of its sides. Composed of two layers of phospholipids that are partly hydrophilic and partly lipophilic, this allows the entrance and exit of both water-soluble and oil-soluble substances—food, waste, and products the cell manufactures as its contribution to the life of the community. Breakage of the membrane docs not easily cause spillage of contents into or out of the cell because the structured water and polymers involved form a different kind of barrier. Embedded in this membrane are various protein molecules that act as portals and pumps that allow material to pass through the membrane, to and fro. These structures seem to be assisted by the gel-like membrane, which also attracts and repels substances (Pollack 2001). The membrane is therefore described as semipermeable.

The cell membrane acts like a "battery" where the energy of the cell is stored. ATP carries energy from the mitochondria to the cell membrane. As the energy is dropped off, the ATP is changed to ADP (one less phosphate) and returned to the mitochondria to pick up energy (when it changes back into ATP). Batteries always have a positive pole and a negative one. The cell membrane is charged positively on the outside and negatively on the inside. This, with anti-binding factors manufactured by matrix polymers, keeps cells from sticking to each other, facilitating the movement of fluids and cells in the ECM.

The cell membrane is capable of wrapping itself around large components and swallowing them, so that the component can be brought into the cell to be broken down by enzymes. This is called *endocytosis*. The same process is used in reverse to expel large components that are no longer needed in the cell; this is called *exocytosis*. However, the majority of cell feeding takes place through portals or channels placed in the membrane. This is the method used by macrophages to consume bacteria and toxins.

Portals in the Cell Membrane: Nutrients and ions enter the cell through microscopic channels or portals in the cell membrane. The larger ones facilitate incoming nutrients, while the smaller ones allow for the passage of ions. The larger channels are composed of proteins bound together by calcium. There are several different kinds using several different mechanisms. Those in the nerves are most famous because they let in calcium, which stimulates muscle contraction, resulting in higher blood pressure. These are the ones that are treated with calcium channel blockers to bring down blood pressure.

At the mouth of some of these channels, nutrients are stacked up for movement into the cytoplasm of the cell. These nutrients have a negative charge that attaches them to positive ions. Calcium is the workhorse among these ions. It can carry up to twenty-two polar compounds, while potassium can only carry eight. Both ions are dragged inside by the rush of the nutrient radicals they are attached to, so that they cannot leave the cell during the assimilative process. However, relieved of their burdens, sodium and calcium are attracted out of the cell by the negative charge on the ECFs. These are also flushed out by electrical charges that require the use of the energy built up in the ADP/ATP cycle. The potassium ions are so large that they end up trapped inside the cell. They are why the ECFs are full of sodium, the intracellular fluids with potassium. Some calcium ions in the cytoplasm bind with phosphate anions to form calcium phosphate, a fairly inert combination. This may be saved for future use or remain in the cell until it is destroyed.

The smaller ion channels operate differently. Each channel restricts passage to specific ions. For instance, a channel barely large enough for a sodium ion to pass through would also allow the smaller magnesium ion to pass, but would deny entry to a large calcium ion and the even larger potassium ion. These passageways also are used to allow the small ions to exit the cell.

The Sodium Pump: It has long been believed that sodium is pumped out of the cell while potassium is retained in a process involving the expenditure of energy from ATP, which is handily present in the cell membrane. It is estimated that about half the energy expended by the cell is bound up in this process. This, however, has been soundly disproven. Richard J. Schmidt explains:

> Gerald Ling carried out some simple experiments . . . as a part of his Ph.D. work. His observations did not fit with the then current understanding of the sodium pump. He writes that he was quietly advised that the sodium pump was a "Holy Cow" and that he should stay away from it. He didn't. His research funding dried up. His research students fled for fear of becoming unemployable. A smear campaign was instigated to blacken his name. (Schmidt, 2003, 857)

Ling's research showed that when ATP production was halted, rather than building up inside the cell, sodium remained in exactly the same balance. In fact, the cell was not inefficiently using half its energy in this "pump." This research was ignored and could not be accounted for until Pollack (2001) suggested that the properties of the structured water complexed in the cell membrane would spontaneously segregate the sodium and potassium. No pump was needed. He too was ignored.

Protoplasm: This word comes from the Greek *protos* (first) and *plasma* (fluid). The protoplasm is the turgid gel that fills the internal space of the cell within the membrane. It is also called the cytoplasm. It is composed of Pollack's structured water, ions, amino acids, proteins, lipids, and large chain sugars. It is believed that the passage of calcium ions in and out of the cytoplasm signals some of the metabolic processes, and it is likely that other electrolytes trigger other processes.

In the more sophisticated, evolved eukaryote cells, there is a central nucleus within the protoplasm. The complex fluid within the nucleus is called the nucleoplasm. However, the nucleus is not actually discontinuous from the protoplasm and is interactive with the cellular signals and substances in which it is surrounded.

Cytoskeleton: This is a loose structural mesh within the cell composed of filaments, microfilaments, and microtubules made out of complex proteins. The cytoskeleton, in combination with the structured water in the protoplasm, controls the life of the cell, maintaining waste removal, cell division, growth, mobility, size, shape, and the uptake of needed material. It is controlled by signals from the matrix and is composed of the same polymers as the ground substance of the matrix; both are generated by enzymes or the Golgi apparatus, so they are contiguous. The centrosome (see below) modifies the polymers under direction from the matrix.

Proteins: The basis of intelligence, communication, and repeatable activities in cells, the proteins divide into two major groups: deoxyribonucleic acid (DNA) and ribonucleic acid (RNA). The former are responsible for long-term information storage and replication or reproduction, while the latter are involved in the ongoing activities of life, including transportation and enzymatic functions.

Organelles: These are tiny organ-like structures that undertake various functions. They include the nucleus, Golgi apparatus, mitochondria, chloroplasts, peroxisomes, and lysosomes.

Centrosome: The centrosome produces microtubules, the key components of the cytoskeleton. It also directs the transportation of molecules through the endoplasmic reticulum and the Golgi apparatus. A single centrosome is present in the cells of animals. It is composed of two centrioles that separate during cell division and help form the mitotic spindle, which is necessary for cellular replication. It operates through the cytoskeleton and protoplasm. However, it is under the control of the electrical charges that operate throughout the extracellular system (ECM) surrounding the cell.

Vacuoles: These are spaces filled with liquid and separated from the protoplasm by a membrane. They can store and transport food, waste, and water. They also transport polymers within the cell or to the membrane for exit into the matrix.

Ribosomes: Ribosomes are made up of a large complex of RNA and protein molecules and are found in both prokaryotes (primitive cells without an organized nucleus) and the more sophisticated, evolved eukaryotes. They act as an assembly line for synthesizing RNA proteins from the amino acids found in the nucleus.

Cell Nucleus: The nucleus is often looked on as the "brain" of the cell, but it really is the reproductive organ. Almost all replication of DNA and synthesis of RNA, the protein chains of the cell that carry information, are undertaken in the nucleus. This includes the chromosomes—the DNA chains responsible for cell replication or reproduction. In eukaryotes, the nucleus is separated from the cytoplasm by a double membrane; in prokaryotes, the nucleus floats in the protoplasm. The addition of a membrane in the eukaryotes protects the DNA and RNA better so that there are fewer mutations.

Chloroplasts: These structures are found only in plants and algae. They capture the sun's energy and, with chlorophyll, manufacture ATP as the energy source for the cell. Plants don't have mitochondria; they have chloroplasts instead.

Endoplasmic Reticulum (ER): The ER is a network that transports molecules that need to be modified to the specific destinations where this can occur. There are two forms, the rough and the smooth ER. The first secretes proteins that assist in this activity, the other does not.

Golgi Apparatus: This structure processes and packages protein and lipid macromolecules that are synthesized within the cell. Macromolecules are the long polymers that are used to construct the cytoskeleton and are extruded from the cell to produce the polymers of the matrix. Five of the six polymers are manufactured by the Golgi apparatus; the sixth (HA) is manufactured by enzymes in the cell protoplasm. This means that HA originated earlier in evolution and is the "primal" ECM polymer. The Golgi apparatus was discovered under the microscope in 1898 by the man whose name it bears, the Italian pathologist Camillo Golgi; its function was not known until recently.

Lysosomes and Peroxisomes: These structures contain enzymes that are so active that they would break down the cell itself where they not contained within a membrane that "damps them down." Lysosomes contain digestive enzymes that break down worn-out organelles, food particles, and engulfed viruses and bacteria. Peroxisomes contain enzymes that rid the cell of toxic peroxides.

Exosomes: These are small bits of protein that resemble viruses. According to conventional theory, they are sent out by cells as signals to other cells when they are under stress from viral attack, but an alternative theory holds that they are the viruses themselves and that what we think of as "viruses" are nothing more than signals sent out by cells reacting to toxins and stress! This theory was brought up by Dr. Thomas S. Cowan and Sally Fallon Morrell in *The Contagion Myth* (2020), during the coronavirus pandemic, and is popular in alternative medicine circles. This is an extremely difficult argument to accept, but it is also difficult to disprove because it has been far more difficult to isolate viruses than is generally known. The authors approve of Arthur Firstenberg's contention that epidemics are associated with electromagnetic frequencies.

Enzymes

Enzymes are found both inside and outside cells. The living organism requires numerous chemical reactions in order to maintain and reproduce itself. These reactions would be very slow were they not catalyzed by little "workbenches" that hold the chemicals so that the reactions can take place rapidly. They are like a shoemaker's last that holds the pieces the shoe is made from. These little "machines" or "molds" are called enzymes.

At the core of every enzyme is an element like boron or magnesium that is set in a protein grid. The reaction catalyzed by the enzyme depends on which element is at its center. The enzyme is not immediately used up by the reaction but remains to be used over and over again when the biochemical reaction it promotes is needed. After a while, the enzyme gets worn out and is broken down by other enzymes. New ones are generated by RNA proteins.

There are three basic classes of enzymes: digestive, metabolic, and dietary. The enzymes in organic matter do all sorts of things, including breaking down the body they are inside. Enzymes are in charge of all biochemical reactions relating to the breakdown and use of food, the elimination of waste products, the repair and building of cells and new tissues, the maintenance of all immune responses, and the breakdown of cancerous cells. Any biological activity we can think of is mediated by enzymes: in fact, thinking itself depends on enzyme catalysts to constantly alter the chemicals that carry codes and messages.

Enzymes work as tireless, highly-skilled workers on a conveyor belt, dismantling, controlling, protecting, destroying, eliminating, reassembling or performing whatever we need in order to exist day and night. After completing their missions and lifespans, enzymes themselves age and are constantly dismantled by other enzymes and then replaced in our bodies. In good health, there is always a new supply of enzymes able and ready to keep on working. (Lopez, Williams, and Mielhke 1994, 9)

The enzymes do indeed work as if on "conveyor belts," but ones that are constantly changing and shifting in activity and position, not fixed conveyor belts, like in our plodding factories. They are constantly acting on foods, wastes, poisons, heat and cold, damp and dry, and the rates and types of reactions. Despite this constant flux, each particular enzyme is a specialist, not a generalist. It acts on only one substance—called a substrate—and in only one way. The enzyme has been likened to a key specific to a certain lock. If even one enzyme is depleted or missing, the body will either have a harder time operating (having to use other, less efficient pathways) or will simply die.

Proper working conditions differ for various enzymes. Some require alkalinity or acidity, some more heat or less. The conditions for one enzyme may oppose conditions needed by another. Enzymes come on-line and go off-line in a constant symphony of purposes and needs that reflect the instant-by-instant requirements of the living organism.

The GRS controls these fluctuations. Flashes of electrical charge zoom up and down the polymers of the matrix into the cell membranes, tripping off enzymatic activities at lightning speed so that the organism is at all times ready and compensating for whatever new environmental influences, foods, or changes are occurring.

The body produces a huge but limited number of enzymes. Edward Howell, a student of the famous naturopathic doctor Henry Lindlahr, theorized that, when the body is no longer able to produce one or several essential for life, health will decline and death will soon occur. This, of course, cannot actually be proven, but it led Howell to point out that the enzymes are therefore equivalent to the vital force in the sense that the extinction of an essential enzyme marks the end of life. It would be better, however, to admit that we don't really know what life is and that we can only see the vital force in its effects— the vital signs that are observed by conventional and unconventional medicine.

Except for a few dozen enzymes in the digestive tract, scientists have not generally been able to substitute man-made enzymes for exhausted enzymes in the body. If this were possible, it would be a therapeutic dream come true. There would be no need for banging around with clumsy drugs. Instead, we could simply introduce a whisper to get our ideas across to the cells.

Actually, we can essentially do this through the matrix. The GRS controls all the organic processes mediated by enzymes; it is the commander in chief and they are the army. Therefore, instead of replacing enzymes or supplementing them, if we can learn to influence them through their control system, then we can make that therapeutic dream come true. And that is what we have been doing for millennia with herbs, acupuncture, massage, cupping, and other methods.

Dr. Howell expounded a doctrine of healing through the consumption of enzymes in food, an idea that has definitely caught on. As he points out, if we consume living foods with enzymes in them, the foods will be partly broken down before our own enzymes will be required. This preserves our limited enzyme production potential. Fermented foods carry comparatively more enzymes than most others.

Each one of us is given a limited supply of bodily enzyme energy at birth. This supply, like the energy supply in your new battery, has to last a lifetime. The faster you use up your enzyme supply, the shorter your life. A great deal of our enzyme energy is wasted haphazardly throughout life. (Howell 1985)

Undoubtedly, this is true in some health conditions. As a general practice, the eating of semicooked and uncooked food will provide enzymes and give the body a rest. However, many herbalists have found that raw food creates its own problems: principally, what would be called a "cold stomach" in traditional Chinese medicine.

If a person has a hot, acidic stomach, the consumption of raw, cold vegetables and fruits, as well as large amounts of water, especially during the meal, will cool off the heat and may benefit the person. I have this kind of stomach and actually have to drink plenty of water during and after a meal. For others, with an average or cold stomach to begin with (meaning poor gastric circulation, innervation, and secretion), this kind of diet further curtails heat and secretion, leading to very low levels of hydrochloric acid and pepsin, resulting in gas, bloating, and serious indigestion. Those with a red tongue need to cool their stomachs; those with a pale tongue need to warm it up.

Mitochondria

One interesting thing that happened in the evolution of cells was that larger ones engulfed smaller ones. The little cells are used as "energy factories" to create energy for themselves as well as for the host cell, which acts as their keeper, feeder, benefactor, and recipient.

These tiny cells are the mitochondria. Their job is to break down glucose to derive energy. The host cell supplies the glucose and the oxygen and takes away the energy, carbon dioxide, and water produced in the chemical reactions in the mitochondrion. The fact that mitochondria were once separate organisms is known because they have a separate genetic code and reproduce separately from the host cell.

?❧ The Krebs or Citric Acid Cycle

The method used by the mitochondria to generate energy is called a cycle because the chemical reactions move in a continuous circle. Each step in the series of reactions requires an organic acid, often named for the plant in which it was originally found (citric acid, malic acid, fumaric acid, aconitic acid, etc.) to advance the operation. The cycle produces nicotinamide adenine dinucleotide (NADH) and other compounds that are used in the cyclic process to create the energy-rich ATP molecule from ADP and inorganic phosphorus. It is remarkable how many of these substances are found in various plants.

ఎ The ADP/ATP Cycle

ATP is used by cells to obtain energy; it's a molecule in which energy is stored in the cell, via bonds between three phosphate atoms. When the energy is released, one phosphate atom is detached to produce the ADP molecule. When the power is dissipated, the ADP picks up new energy, in the form of an extra phosphate, becoming a new ATP molecule. This chemical change is produced in the mitochondria, due to the citric acid cycle. Extra ATP is stored in the cell membrane, which operates like a battery (positive on the outside and negative on the inside).

ఎ Lactic Acid

If not enough oxygen is present to break down all the glucose in the Krebs cycle, the cell switches to a process called *glycolysis* or *glycosylation* to break it down. This generates energy, but also lactic acid. That is why, when we exercise above the normal level, we can't get enough oxygen and lactic acid builds up, causing aches in the muscles being used.

Red blood cells can't use the Krebs cycle because they are carrying oxygen molecules that would tend to become reactive in the presence of the substances in the cycle. Instead, the red blood cell makes itself a low maintenance level of energy from glycosylation with lactic acid. Red blood cells are, therefore, barely living cells with a short life span of about seventy days.

If too much lactic acid builds up in regular cells, it would eventually cause them to deteriorate. Calcium acts as a buffer, picking up lactic acid and keeping it out of circulation.

As mentioned previously, cancer cells use this more primitive form of energy generation to support themselves. "Glycosylation Defining Cancer Malignancy: New Wine in an Old Bottle," by Senitiroh Hakomori (2002) points out the importance of this.

> Aberrant glycosylation occurs in essentially all types of experimental and human cancers, as has been observed for over 35 years, and many glycosyl epitopes constitute tumor-associated antigens. A long-standing debate is whether aberrant glycosylation is a result or a cause of cancer. Many recent studies indicate that some, if not all, aberrant glycosylation is a result of initial oncogenic transformation, as well as a key event in induction of invasion and metastasis. Glycosylation promoting or inhibiting tumor cell invasion and metastasis is of crucial importance in current cancer research. Nevertheless, this area of study has received little attention from most cell biologists involved in cancer research, mainly because structural and functional concepts of glycosylation in cancer are more difficult to understand than the functional role of certain proteins and their genes in defining cancer cell phenotypes.

The relationship between cancer and glycosylation was first described by Dr. Otto Warburg (1883–1970), a medical doctor and physiologist who would later be awarded the Nobel Peace Prize for his work in isolating a respiratory enzyme. He looked into the sudden upsurge of cancer in the early twentieth century and found that cancer cells were using glycolysis while most healthy cells were not. This is known as the "Warburg Effect." Because he attributed the sudden rise in cancer to chemical toxins that had been introduced into the environment in the preceding decades, this work was largely ignored by conventional medicine. As for Warburg himself: he retired to an acre and tended his organic garden for the rest of his long life. His work is only now coming to be appreciated (Firstenberg 2016).

Because glycosylation causes an increase in lactic acid, it has been presumed by the lay public that cancer would be defeated by consumption of alkaline food. Conventional science, on the other hand, has long argued that this type of thinking is incorrect since the body as a whole is buffered to maintain a pH between 7.35 and 7.45. This, first of all, turns out not to be true for the matrix, and second, turns out not to be true in the microenvironment immediately surrounding cancer cells. A disturbed pH is also found in diabetes. Therefore, "extracellular acidity has been shown to be relevant" to the origin of these diseases. However, "targeting acidity and defining the mechanisms driving acidity are still nascent areas of investigation" (Gillies, Pilot, Marunaka, and Fais 2019).

Although eating alkaline and organic foods are popular approaches to cancer prevention, the reduction in caloric intake holds the greatest potential for reducing acid waste products affecting both cancer and diabetes because it directly increases oxidation, while reducing glycosylation. There is now research supporting the ketogenic diet in this regard (Tran, Lee, Kim, Kong, Gong, Kwon, Park, Kim, and Park 2020).

The ketogenic diet is a high-fat, low-carb, protein-adequate diet that causes the body to burn fats rather than carbs. It is officially used in medicine to treat hard-to-control epilepsy in children, but it is used in alternative medicine for weight loss, insulin resistant diabetes (since it reduces carbohydrates), hard-to-treat inflammatory conditions, and other conditions.

৯৬ Purine Signaling Network

This is a special signaling system that works through molecules associated with the mitochondria such as ADP and ATP. The reason the mitochondria are involved is that the response and memory of the stressor are recorded in the metabolism of the cell. These "purinergic" signals move inside cells and through the adjoining matrix to nearby cells. Purinergic receptors are among some of the most common in the biological world.

൞ Cell Danger Response

This new theory has largely been propounded by Robert Naviaux, from whom I have derived much of the following account (Naviaux 2019).

The cell danger response (CDR), dependent largely on the mitochondria, is a reaction to stress in the cell that occurs when threats exceed the ability of the cell to maintain homeostasis. It can be triggered by chemical, physical, or biological stressors, and it appears that the mitochondria shift their action from energy production through the Krebs cycle to membrane protection. The event is therefore registered in a metabolic response and stored in a metabolic memory bank.

When stressors attack the cell, a mismatch results between the amount of energy, resources, and capabilities available to the cell and the amount required to keep homeostasis in balance. Changes occur in electron flow, oxidation, and reduction. This changes membrane fluidity, lipid balance, energy availability, carbon and sulfur availability, protein management, vitamin use, and many other factors.

A response in the mitochondria occurs in the "first wave" of danger signaling. There are changes in the release of ATP and ADP, the actions of free radicals and intermediate molecules in the Krebs cycle, and oxidation. These changes can be stepped up through the purinergic signaling—a "second wave."

Naviaux notes, "After the danger has been eliminated or neutralized, a choreographed sequence of anti-inflammatory and regenerative pathways is activated to reverse the CDR and to heal" (Naviaux 2014). If the CDR persists, the metabolism of the whole body will be disturbed, the gut microbiome changed, and the coordination of organ systems impaired. Chronic disease will appear, and a person's behavior can even change.

Normally, when the threat passes, the mitochondria go through three distinct phases in the process of their return to normal function. Chronic disease can manifest if the mitochondria get stuck in any of these three phases, with the disease process being somewhat particular to the phase where the CDR gets stuck.

Memories of past stress encounters are stored in a kind of "metabolic memory bank" in the cell and mitochrondrion. This produces an increase in the reserve capacity to face stressors in the future.

CDR and the magnified form induced by the purinergic life-threatening response are ultimately controlled by centers in the brainstem. Integration of the whole body metabolic response occurs in the brainstem. This is a "prerequisite" for normal brain, motor, sensory, social, and speech activities.

An understanding of the CDR permits us to reframe old concepts of pathogenesis for a broad array of chronic, developmental, autoimmune, and degenerative disorders. These disorders include autism spectrum disorders (ASD); attention deficit hyperactivity disorder (ADHD); asthma; atopy; gluten and many other food and chemical sensitivity syndromes; emphysema; Tourette's syndrome; bipolar disorder; schizophrenia; post-traumatic stress disorder (PTSD); chronic traumatic encephalopathy (CTE); traumatic brain injury (TBI); epilepsy; suicidal ideation; organ transplant biology; diabetes; kidney, liver, and heart disease; cancer; Alzheimer's and Parkinson's diseases; and autoimmune disorders like lupus, rheumatoid arthritis, multiple sclerosis, and primary sclerosing cholangitis (Naviaux 2014).

CELL DEATH

When a cell has reached the natural conclusion of its life cycle, it does not just rot, like a dead animal, but undergoes an intentional self-destruction called *apoptosis,* during which it shrinks and fragments into pieces. These are then consumed by macrophages, which are in turn consumed as they age and decline by other phagocytic cells. Apoptosis and phagocytosis keep the matrix clean and prevent mutated cells from multiplying—preventing cancer, in other words.

Cells can also deteriorate and die prematurely due to infections or toxins. This results in necrosis: the cell's internal structure shrinks and detaches from its external membrane, causing the membrane to burst and disintegrate. The cell blows apart, and the pieces spread through the matrix. The mess is cleaned up by macrophages that are suddenly produced in great number—a high white blood cell count, as biomedicine would say—to meet the challenge of toxicity and infection by bacteria feeding off the debris.

COMPARTMENTALIZATION OF THE MATRIX

The organs or tissues of the body are separated into compartments by serous membranes generated by epithelial cells, usually with a basement membrane or interstitium between the membrane and the matrix. Signals and interstitial fluids can cross these membranes, but the ground substance generally remains where it is, on one side or the other.

The composition of the matrix is consistent throughout the organism—water, proteins, polysaccharides—but each different tissue has a matrix with a composition unique to itself. This is generated "through a dynamic and reciprocal, biochemical and biophysical dialogue" (Frantz, Stewart, and Weaver 2010) that is ongoing while the tissue and its matrix are developing, both in utero and throughout life. Thus, the composition of the local ECM is tissue specific and varies throughout the organism.

The ECM generates the biochemical and mechanical properties of each organ, such as its tensile and compressive strength and elasticity, and also mediates protection by a buffering action that maintains extracellular homeostasis and water retention. (Frantz, Stewart, and Weaver 2010)

In other words, it's the "knitting" that makes each tissue and organ unique, and there can be wide differences between the strength and efficiency of different organs and tissues within the same organism. The overall constitution of the person, so to speak, does not completely dominate in local areas, so that there can be significant differences from organ to organ. This accounts for a phenomena that is widely recognized by professional medical practitioners and the public alike: one person has a strong stomach and another does not, or a person is strong throughout but has, say, a weak heart, so that the powerful athlete suddenly falls dead.

The matrix directs the "essential morphological organization and physiological function" in the tissue "by binding growth factors (GFs) and interacting with cell-surface receptors" (Frantz, Stewart, and Weaver 2010) to send signals into the cells or tissues that control gene transcription (DNA and RNA functions), while at the same time influencing the tissue by matrix flexibility. Any of these factors—lack of control of gene transcription, lack of flexibility in the matrix, and high levels of growth factors—if out of balance, can cause cancer. Thus, a person who is entirely well, has good genetics, eats sensibly, and exercises can fall prey to a terrible cancer that seemingly descends on them out of nowhere. It is not too much to say that we must grade our matrix as the seedbed of our lifelong health.

Organ Specificity

Not only is each tissue and organ unique, to some extent, from the organism as a whole, but we also have to acknowledge a second corollary: a natural level of organization and self-regulation occurs within the organism at the level of tissues and organs. As we have seen, the matrix is differentiated in each organ compartment. So once again, it is not the individual cell that should be looked upon as a key to organization and regulation in the body, but the matrix or whole organization and the natural compartments within the matrix, the organs. Separate functions, associated with these organs and with tissues, should also be considered here.

This conforms to a widely held tenant of traditional, natural, and alternative medicine that is often assumed but not explained. In complementary and alternative medicine, we often treat the tissue or organ as a whole rather than attending to the condition of the cells or even to the whole organism. This reflects the natural wear and tear on a local area of the body that is produced by eating irritating food, or nonfibrous food, or working in a particular environment. Indeed, this is what average people often say: "My stomach is weak," "Uncle Joe's lungs are strong," "I've got thin blood," and so on. This type of information, shared during an intake with a holistic practitioner, is meaningful in that arena, but it is often meaningless when shared with a medical professional, who is taught to adhere strictly to what the medical tests report, without direct interaction between the practitioner and the patient.

Not only does the alternative practitioner seek to view and treat the person as a whole, but he or she also treats the local tissues and organs as independent spheres to some extent, each one a whole to itself, as it were, within the greater economy of the whole organism.

This orientation is visible in just about every school of alternative medicine known and practiced. We certainly see it in traditional Chinese medicine, which usually treats the *zangfu* (organs and bowels) or sometimes the tissue (qi, blood, fluids). It is an axiom of Western herbalism as well, with its "liver remedies" and "blood purifiers." It is true of classical osteopathy, which treats the local distribution of the blood, that is to say, local areas, and of traditional chiropractic, which assigns organs to the autonomic ganglia along the spine. It is true of Greek medicine and the "organopathy" of homeopathy.

This idea can also be justified from a pharmacological standpoint. I used to talk about organ specificity with herbalist David Hoffmann. One year he said, "I've finally figured out the pharmacological justification for organ specificity in herbs." He reminded me that adrenergic and cholinergic effects were originally defined by the action of plants such as *Atropa belladonna*. In the same manner, other medicinal plants could be used to define actions of organs and their treatment.

MOTHER, BABY, AND MATRIX

I had not given thought to the theme of the development of an individual's matrix during the fetal epoch and babyhood, but this was the subject of meditation by herbalist Michelle Carnochan of Australia, who gave me permission to share her thoughts.

Back in the day, during a semester of nutritional biochemistry, I learned that babies are born with purposefully designed "leaky guts." That is, their gut membrane is full of tiny little holes. This doesn't seal up until the appearance of the first teeth. There's an ingenious reason for this. Mother's breast milk is full of proteins including antibodies and other immunity-founding components, as well as the macronutrients—fat, carbs, and protein. The "leaky gut" of the baby allows these large proteins to move through and start establishing a good foundation for the immune system. Different microflora species, as well the food they need, are also found in breast milk, and this—along with the flora received during the normal birth process—helps to establish the baby's own gut microbiome.

My understanding from this is that the emergence of the teeth now signals that, along with this sealing of the gut membrane, the baby is now ready for solids and other foreign proteins—found in other animal products and grains in particular. Introduction of these prior to this milestone confuses the fledgling immune system and sets up an immune response, which if coupled with other foreign intrusions (such as formaldehyde, aluminum, mercury, and recombinant DNA from bovine, porcine, simian, and aborted human fetal tissue), results in the development of allergies and food intolerances. But in learning about the ECM I've now come to a slightly more developed understanding. . . .

Anyway, now I have to wonder, as I examine breast milk more closely: yes, it seems to be the same consistency as ECM fluid. Indeed most secretions in and from the body are composed of this fluid. With this in mind, I then have to wonder whether the importance of breast milk lies not so much in the immune proteins, etc., that it provides (although the love, comfort, and nutritional nourishment is paramount), does it—as an extension of the mother's matrix—actually entrain the baby's matrix? (Such as how we see the mother's heart entrain the baby's to beat at a regular rhythm, or the mother's breathing patterns entrain the baby's.) This speaks to the instinct (now often over-ridden) to carry our newborns around, or sleep next to them, keeping them close to our hearts.

When we introduce milk from another animal before the appropriate time, does the baby's body instead recognize that this matrix material simply does not carry the same "vibe" as the mother's matrix? After all, as I write this I have to conclude that amniotic fluid also has its origins in the matrix fluid, and given that the baby has spent some 40 weeks being bathed in this very personal imprint of his or her mother, I suspect that the similarities would be instantly recognized—at least on a sub-conscious or instinctive level [if not an immune level].

This is important, because if we understand the incredible significance of this matrix (interestingly, from the Latin—also meaning "mother"), on the regulation of our bodies and our overall health, then surely we should come to a greater appreciation of how important this liquid gold of human breast milk is to our children. (Michelle Carnochan, personal communication)

These thoughts perhaps make the idea of the ECM more intimate and personal.

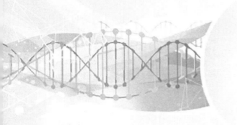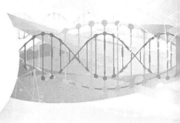

6

The In-Mix-Out of the Matrix
Basis for Holistic Treatment

So you've got the in-mix-out, and when you think of that, you've got a simplification of the whole business of disease. . . . The body takes in certain raw materials; it works over them; then it throws out the waste.

DR. WILLIAM M. DAVIDSON (1979, 31)

The basic patterns of physiological activity in a living organism can be reduced to a simple formula: in-mix-out. All functions, organs, and systems in the body function according to this simple model, but *if ever there were a single system that required this sort of generalization as the foundation for physiological study, it would be the matrix.* In holism, we seek to understand how all the parts come together into whole functional units, and this is how we must look at the matrix to develop holistic methods of treatment.

In this chapter, therefore, we quote only holistic physicians and practitioners because they are the only ones who have generated any kind of holistic treatment of the matrix. Dr. William Davidson was a medical astrologer: if there is any group of people who can hone down processes into patterns and name them, it is the astrologers.

BOUNDARIES OF THE MATRIX

In order to visualize or treat the in-mix-out, we need to establish the boundaries of the matrix. This would be the capillary wall, where the contents of the matrix flow *in* from the blood, the cell membranes that mark one end of the matrix, and the lymphatic capillaries that take *out* the excess and garbage. Between this lies the *mix* that occurs in the matrix and the cells themselves: the ongoing functions of metabolism that require input from the blood and export through the lymphatics.

Pischinger considered the "capillary-matrix-cell" to be the basic unit of functional activity in the body. In his lifetime, this would have included the lymphatic capillaries, which were thought of as part of the circulatory system. Now, however, we think of them in association with the immune system. Pischinger conceived the basic functional unit of the body to be the area and activities largely controlled by the GRS. We have seen how the GRS can actually help choose what comes into the matrix, even differing the selection from one compartment to another. In addition, the immune cells stationed just inside the matrix from the capillary bed also control what gets into the matrix. The matrix naturally presses contents into the lymphatic capillaries for removal. There is some slight push back from the capillary bed, the cell, and the lymphatic ducts, especially if there is disease (microbiomes, purine cell signals, electrolyte imbalances, lymphatic stagnation, etc.), but Pischinger's thesis is clearly appropriate.

THE PATHOLOGY AND THERAPY OF THE IN-MIX-OUT

Long before the ECM was considered to have any real value, and long before the discovery of the GRS, various practitioners developed therapeutic methods for dealing with the matrix, even though it was ignored, unnamed, or unknown to conventional medicine. Several different "schools" can be traced. The Viennese had never given up on the teachings of Carl von Rokitansky, so Harmut Heine speaks of four generations of therapeutic success in Vienna, based on the concept of the importance of the circulation and the matrix (Pischinger 1991). Then there were the French, whose tradition included Marie Françoise Xavier Bichat, Claude Bernard, and A. Béchamp. This led to the important work of Marguerite Maury in the field of aromatherapy. In North America, Walter Cannon's work on the homeostasis of the milieu intérieur and Hans Selye's work on stress were both accepted by conventional medicine and are an important part of modern biomedicine. Most colorful of all would be the Salt Lake City naturopath Samuel West, who made the treatment of the space between the cells (for him it still had no name) almost a fundamentalist religious dogma.

I am not sure if there are more undercurrents and connections than I am aware of between these people. Maury (1895–1968) was trained as a nurse in Vienna, where the influence of Rokitansky was palpable; later, she moved to Paris and became a medical doctor. At that time, women could not advance into the medical fraternity in Austria. Maury followed Bichat's theory of the lacunary system, which, as we have seen, is basically an early and accurate conception of the ECM. She resuscitated aromatherapy, which she saw as having a special relationship with the extracellular space through the diffusion of odiferous scents from the skin.

One could hardly find two practitioners with less in common than Maury and West, yet their basic ideas about the matrix were essentially the same. Either they came up with these ideas independently and intuitively or there was some link between them. Possibly, this was through the International Society of Lymphologists, of which West often spoke.

Marguerite Maury

Maury resuscitated aromatherapy by providing medical explanations based on the work of Bichat, whose lacunary system describes the matrix. "There is a continual exchange between the blood, the lymph and the lacunary liquid," all of which circulate in their own sphere, the blood passing to what she calls the "lacunary centre" and from there to the lymph and back into the circulatory system (Maury 1996, 23).

In addition, Maury also adopted the perspective of Dr. Alexandre Zalmanoff (1895–1968), who emphasized the flexibility, dilation, contraction, and regulatory and immune effects of the capillary bed. I've already written a chapter about the importance of the circulatory system in *Traditional Western Herbalism and Pulse Evaluation: A Conversation* (Wood, Bonaldo, and Light 2016), so we will not cover that subject here.

The matrix is subject to upsets caused by all sorts of stressors. Homeostasis fluctuates due to changes in the environment, but for the dial to be reset on a chronic pathological condition, it needs to be overwhelmed by something so strong that it cannot return to homeostatic balance. This results in we what we now call allostasis—an altered balance of bodily function following disease. Therefore, Maury concluded that the major pathological influence that really impacts the lacunary system is "shock," as she called it, or overwhelming change, either physical or psychological.

This is a very significant observation because real physiological shock causes the pathological exudation of blood cells, blood proteins, and plasma into the matrix. "These shocks produce a kind of plastic exudation," explains Maury (1996, 23), so that, "one might say that the blood bleeds in the tissues," that is, the matrix. Many changes result from this occurrence, of which Maury lists the following:

Inhibition of cell division
Invasion of healthy tissues by connective tissue
Cellulitis, or the collection in the ECM of "vitiated organic liquid"
Thickening of the skin due to capillary congestion
Irritation of the skin due to excessive capillary sanguification
Wrinkling of the skin (lack of feeding via the capillaries)
Insensate and inactive skin, no longer resistant to the weather and
    ill-treatment

Slackening of facial and other muscles, resulting in a transformation of appearance (Maury 1996, 22, 24)

We saw virtually all of these factors associated with injury to the matrix in chapter 4, which covered wound healing.

Marguerite Maury's Guide to Aromatherapy does not contain a lot of specific information about the therapeutic treatment of the matrix, but she gives a valuable overview of the properties of essential oils in regard to their abilities to move into the matrix. She grades them as (1) resins, (2) medium-density essential oils, and (3) highly volatile oils:

Very heavy resin-bearing substances and rather dense essential oils apply in general to the purely vegetable and cellular domain; here the quality of the tissues is influenced and also the assimilation of foods.

Essential oils of average tonality influence above all the function. The influence extends to the vago-sympathetic system and orders the functional rhythm.

The third category, the very fluid oils of swift and almost incisive evaporation, seem to enter into direct contact with that part of the brain which is not the seat of consciousness. Moreover, this last category of essential oils penetrates with the greatest ease into the extra-cellular liquids. (Maury 1995, 97)

In other words, resins act on the tissues and tissue feeding, medium-density essential oils on the functions of the organs and their function rate, and highly volatile oils penetrate deeply into the organism. Her statement about the influence on the "part of the brain which is not the seat of consciousness," is explained in the following comment:

Odoriferous matter reaches the regions of the brain which are not under conscious control; its perception affects our psychic life and transforms our predispositions. (Maury 1996, 92)

Knowing these differences helps not only in therapeutic application of these agents but also in their formulation.

> The heaviest part retains and slows down the pervasive [diffusive] part which would be too swift were it allowed to act on its own. The whole is united by the moderation of the medium part, the result being that when the whole compound penetrates the extra-cellular liquids, the two elements, the slow and the moderated, are encouraged by a swift part, which is found to be the most voluminous. . . . The two heavy elements determine that the diffusion operates gently and at a rate suitable to the body. (Maury 1996, 97)

One should not get the impression that these essential oils and resins alone act on the matrix; many other medicinal substances are also active, especially mucilage, the particles of which are allied to the matrix polymers. At any rate, these observations may serve as guidelines for applying herbal agents to the matrix.

Maury does not give a lot of specific indications for essential oils. She does say that "essence of violet leaves is paramount in dissolving rheumatic toxins; it is therefore suitable for re-establishing a certain elasticity of the tissues and muscles" (Maury 1996, 104). As it happens, the leaves of the Violet are mucilaginous and moistening. Lemongrass dispels and absorbs "dead cells and their waste" to eliminate tumors. Sandalwood "opens the renal sluices" and dispels "melancholic humors" (Maury 1995, 104–5). For a more detailed treatment of essential oils in relation to herbalism see *Principles of Holistic Therapy with Herbal Essences* (Gümbel 1993).

Samuel West

Samuel West (1934–2002) was a naturopath in the generation of Bernard Jensen, John Bastyr, and John Christopher. He lived and practiced in Salt Lake City. He simplified natural healing down to a single concept: flush the fluids in and out of the compartment between the capillary bed, the cell membranes, and the lymphatic capillaries. West didn't have a name for this compartment, but of course we recognize it as the ECM. He didn't use the terminology "in-mix-out," but he would have agreed with it implicitly. He recognized, like Maury, that proteins entering the matrix would damage the compartment on one end and that poor lymphatic drainage would stop up the matrix at the other end. This led West to propose a universal method of treatment: vegetarianism (to reduce proteins) and the use of a small trampoline ("lymphaciser") to move the lymph. This idea is laudable for its simplicity and universality, but West did not oppose the use of other methods of holistic treatment that would contribute to the healing of the compartment between the cells.

West tells us how he made the intuitive leap to his understanding from a simple statement in a medical book. In the fifth edition of the *Textbook of Medical Physiology,* Dr. Arthur C. Guyton, wrote:

> The lymphatic system represents an accessory route by which fluids can flow from the interstitial spaces back to the blood. And, most important of all, the lymphatics can carry proteins and large particulate matter away from the tissue spaces, neither of which can be removed by absorption directly into the blood capillary. We shall see that this removal of proteins from the interstitial spaces is an absolutely essential function without which we would die within about twenty four hours. (Guyton 1976, 397)

West understood from this the importance of keeping the compartment of interstitial fluids around the cells in good health and how to accomplish this by limiting the uptake of proteins into the matrix and keeping the lymphatics clean and flowing.

When I read this, I was reminded of a statement by my friend Dennis Anderson, a holistic healer in Mondovi, Wisconsin. Born a farmer, Dennis said, "The best exercise for the lymphatics is horseback riding." I have always used herbs for this work. West did not, in fact, oppose any method—massage, homeopathy, herbalism—that would get the lymphatics moving. Dennis also advocates or uses all these techniques.

Like Maury, West realized that shock caused the capillaries to dump blood proteins and cells into the matrix. His suggestion of vegetarianism is congruent with the recommendation of Pischinger (1991, 28): "Deposits of metabolic waste . . . can be worked-off with protein fasting."

West was a member of the International Society of Lymphologists—mostly medical doctors and researchers—a group that must have been familiar with the work of Pischinger, Heine, and others in developing the concept of the ECM and GRS. However, his teachings, writings, and illustrations refer to nothing more complicated than the idea of a space full of water between the blood capillaries, the cells, and the lymphatic drain ways.

West's practice and teaching methods took on a typically American variation. One of his students, herbalist Steven Horne, remembers West from the early 1980s.

> I spent a full year working with Dr. C. Samuel West and his International Academy of Lymphology. For those of you who never met Dr. West, he was a dynamic crusader determined to spread the word about the "gospel" of lymphology. . . . His classes were like revival meetings dedicated to spreading the "good word" about healing the body via the lymphatic system. He is best-known for his promotion of "lymphasing" or rebound exercise on a mini-trampoline. (Horne 2009)

West's enthusiasm manifested in another burning interest: he was a tax protester who fought the federal income tax. This led to his death in a freak accident at the Federal Courthouse in Salt Lake City in 2002. After arguing his case before the judge, he turned and grasped a handrail that had recently been "repaired." The screws had not been replaced, the rail gave way, and he fell, smashing his head on a step and dying several weeks later. While he was semiconscious, he was, as his family reported, tortured by medical procedures he would never have approved of. The tax judgment went against him.

In his therapeutic teachings, West pointed out that in a healthy condition of what we call the matrix, there is only enough fluid to fill the spaces around the cells, and no more. This water has a negative pressure with the capillary bed and cells pressing in on it. However, if debris builds up in the matrix, then water will become trapped, and this will lead to a puffed-up condition in which the pressure in the matrix is higher and the capillaries can't dump off metabolites and oxygen, the cells can't dump their garbage or get fed, and the lymphatics will be congested. There is also an excess of sodium, since sodium soaks up water. This is the basic condition in essential hypertension, in which there is an excess of sodium in the matrix with a pressure exerted outward against the capillary bed, causing high blood pressure.

Modern medicine sees this as a problem of sodium buildup to be controlled by a low-sodium diet, calcium channel blockers, and diuretics, but this may put the cart before the horse: the sodium may be building up due to the water retention caused by local inflammation and waste-product buildup, overfeeding, or low lymphatic function. Low potassium is also especially damaging.

Excess water and waste buildup trigger self-cleansing processes that are inflammatory in nature. Both acute and chronic inflammation can overwhelm the lymphatic drainage out of the matrix, often forcing it to become the weak link in the whole system. The endothelial gaps in the lymphatic capillaries close if there is inflammation in the ECM. This is called lymphadenitis or lymph endothelial gap stasis. When the gaps are open and all other factors are in place, the matrix compartment is beautifully cleansed.

Samuel West's ideas are laid out in his book *Golden Seven Plus One* (1981).

THE DETAILS OF "IN"

The distribution of the blood, via the shunting to and fro of the circulation by the arterioles, is considered by many holistic practitioners to be either the basis of local indispositions of health or to accompany these local changes.

We cannot say that this is an age-old medical model because it was only in 1628 that the circulation of the blood became known through the work of William Harvey. However, in the nineteenth century, the basic mechanics of the distribution of the circulation were known, at least in a nice, workable outline. It was at this time that the idea of "equalizing the circulation" was a guiding light in conventional, botanical, osteopathic, and Rokitansky's medicine.

Modern medicine, outside of Germany and parts of Europe, does not largely consider the subject of circulatory distribution, but biomedicine does acknowledge diseases of the capillary bed. The important ones are capillary fragility and lack of permeability. These are marked by the appearance of bruises, varicosities, spider veins, or hemorrhoids—showing easy congestion, vessel breakage, and permeability. These may be related to the larger context of circulatory disorder that holistic practitioners are looking for.

The Capillary Bed

The matrix is fed by the terminal vessels of the cardiovascular system, the capillaries. To deal with environmental and internal stressors, the body directs blood to or away from certain areas. The observation of this fact led to Rokitansky's insistence on the importance of the circulation as a diagnostic and therapeutic tool in medicine, the origin of osteopathy, proof of the osteopathic premise by Irvin Korr, and the widespread monitoring of the skin (color, texture, moisture) in traditional medicine. This orientation is found everywhere from the Native American sweat lodge to Chinese herbalism to the great herbal traditions of nineteenth-century America.

To get a specific measurement of capillary health, medical tests were developed in the early twentieth century based on temporary use of the tourniquet. After a length of time, the tourniquet is released and the number of petechiae (tiny bruises) are counted.

This is not a practice I plan to adopt. Of more use to the holistic practitioner is a simple eyeball examination of the complexion. The presence of blue in any shade is an indication for what the Chinese call "stagnant blood" or "congealed blood." This complexion is associated with local bruises (which are usually bluish) but also with system-wide constitutional tendencies. The blue color could be interpreted either as an excess of blood remaining on the venous side of the circulation, capillary fragility, or a low-grade, widespread coagulative tendency of the blood. As the condition gets worse, there will be bleeding from outlets (nose, rectum) as well as coagulation, since there are not enough platelets where they are needed. I have seen coagulation with bleeding several times.

One can determine some parameters of capillary and circulatory health just by looking in the right places on the skin. Look at the pads of the palms. If they are reddish, the blood is backing up in the capillaries. If one indents the pad with the fingertip, takes it away, and the area takes a while—one to three seconds—for color to come back into the pad, the indication is that blood is taking a good bit of time to flow back into the capillary bed. If there is redness on the back of the hand and pallor occurs after pressure, the indication is also stronger because the capillary bed is not as thick here as on the pads of the palm. I talked to a hospice doctor who also used this informal test to determine the health of her patients. If the blanching after the finger was taken away lasted as long as three seconds, the patient was probably soon to pass on. In a younger person, this is not an indication of mortality but of capillary inflammation making the reentry of blood slow, or low blood pressure. In most healthy people, the amount of time it takes for the blood to flow back varies from day to day. In the sanguine temperament, the full redness of the cheeks of the face and the palms is normal but may still indicate health tendencies.

If the pad of the palm or the backside of the hand is naturally red or reddens shortly after pressure, we know there is a certain amount of peripheral fullness, histaminic irritation, immune excess, or inflammation in the capillary bed. We can see why this test would indicate inflammation in the capillary bed. This can occur from two opposite problems. In the first instance, the engorgement may be caused by resistance to the red blood cells, which are larger than the capillary diameter, as they pass through the vessel. This might be due to inflammation of the membranes of the capillaries from heat, irritation, overactivity of the immune system, or poor quality of lipids in the diet causing irritable cell membranes. This would cause resistance against the outward circulation, resulting in high blood pressure. In the second instance, the cause would be low blood pressure from the heart and arteries not pushing outwardly so strongly. This is particularly what the hospice doctor was finding. I also find this a good indication for low blood pressure, but my clients are not as sick.

In cases of either high or low blood pressure, the remedies are the same, interestingly. This is a good indicator for Hawthorn and Wild Cherry bark, so I suppose it to be due to problems with lipids in the blood vessels (Hawthorn) or histaminic irritation (Cherry). Low blood pressure is as much an indicator for Hawthorn as high. If the padding is red with patches of deep red, the indication is for Rose Hips or Rose Petals and the inflammation is moving deeper. If there is mottling on the arm (red, blue, white), Elder Flower is often indicated.

We can also look at the tongue for indications. If the outer edge is red, pale, swollen, tooth-marked, damp, or dry compared with the center of the tongue, there is a difference in circulation between the periphery and the central circulation. Red on the sides and blue in the center is a good indication for Yarrow, which I have verified maybe a hundred times. It indicates heat in the periphery and blood stagnation in the center. Yarrow may also be indicated if the edges of the tongue are pale and the center is red, or vice versa. If the edges of the tongue are swollen and scalloped, this is usually taken as evidence of "spleen deficiency" in traditional Chinese medicine or poor assimilation. I take it as a sign of swollen, damp mucous membranes, which is saying the same thing since "spleen qi holds up the tissues" to prevent relaxation and prolapse. But this is also an indication of problems with the peripheral circulation. Anytime the tongue is carmine red, there is capillary engorgement and irritation, and the usual call is for cooling remedies. Linden Flower and Yellow Dock Root are also to be considered here.

The pulse is a window looking into the heart, cardiovascular system, and capillary bed. One can feel the resistance against the outward flow or the weakness of the outward circulation. (It must be remembered that the capillaries literally pull in the blood; they are not just passive, so the problem may be in the center or the circumference.) We won't go into the topic here, because it is so complicated: see *Traditional Western Herbalism and Pulse Evaluation: A Conversation* (Wood, Bonaldo, and Light 2016).

These observations can be made on people of various races. They actually sometimes show the disharmony between a race of people and the environment they are living in. For instance, the redness (and yellowness) on the back of the hand or the palm is very common, in my experience, in White people in Arizona, California, and Australia.

I find that I get the best results in healing *overall* when I treat the circulatory condition and see changes in the color of the tongue and complexion and qualities of the pulse. These changes reflect the overall condition of the person as well as the local manifestations.

When there is stagnant or congealed blood, to use the Chinese expression, we have a different set of indications. We look for blue in the tongue or complexion and choppiness (randomness) in the beat (not heartbeat) of the pulse. The following specific indications help to differentiate cases: Yarrow, Arnica, Safflower oil (red and blue bruise showing inflammation); the homeopathics Carbo vegetabilis and Carbo animalis (lingering blue and yellow coloration of the bruise); Angelica (blue, green, gray, and yellow coloration around the veins, or black/blue veins under the tongue); Madder (*Rubia tinctoria*) and Sage (*Salvia officinalis, S. miltorrhiza*) (blue and gray complexion of skin or tongue); Sassafras (blue and black contusions and complexion); homeopathic Conium (Poison Hemlock) (black contusions of the elderly); Elder Flower (blue and swollen pale around a joint); and Red Root (I don't know the differentials).

Coagulation of the blood was a characteristic symptom during the COVID pandemic. In the experience of many herbalists, the medicines that ameliorated the severity of the symptoms were warming and drying (Angelica, Lomatium, Osha, Cinnamon, Rosemary, Yarrow, Cayenne, Bayberry, Yerba Mansa, Onion syrup, Garlic, etc.). These thin the blood, increase peripheral circulation (which reduces blood pressure), and thin and usually promote expectoration of mucus.

Sometimes we need to increase capillary permeability, mostly to move fluids and minerals. To increase capillary permeability, I use the great American Indian medicine Gravel Root (*Eupatorium purpureum*). This medicinal agent is indicated in stiffness due to calcification and lack of lubrication in the muscles and tissues. It increases capillary profusion. Yarrow also seems to have a like effect, though it is probably achieved by increasing peripheral circulation, not just increasing profusion of blood from the capillaries.

Herbalist Dawn Gates, a longtime cardiac and hospital nurse who has been watching patients and MRIs and facial and skin tones and indications for years, taught us that the lower tip of the heart is susceptible to decreasing capillary profusion. This explained to me why I had one client who felt Gravel Root revived her failing heart and another who felt the same way after we added Yarrow to her Hawthorn (one part to three).

The effect of Gravel Root on opening the capillaries of the blood and lymph circulation was noted by several herbalists in addition to myself: Richard Riordan, of Pasadena, and Sondra Boyd, a Tsalagi medicine woman who drew on ancient traditions as well as experience. Richard and I were just lucky to note this action.

Varicosities and hemorrhoids indicate venous ill-health and are treatable by a range of old, traditional astringents such as Horse Chestnut, Collinsonia, Witch Hazel, Yarrow (red and blue skin color, spider veins, bleeding hemorrhoids), and Oak bark (nasty, big varicosities with blue, black, and yellow discoloration around them).

An important herb here is Horsetail, which is not an astringent. It seems to work differently: increasing strength through mineralization. It is high in silicon, a structural element, although there is only a small amount of this mineral available in the hard stalks. I know several practitioners who rely on this one remedy, claiming it is that specific for varicosities.

As soon as we cross over the capillary bed into the matrix, we find ourselves in the presence of little agents of immunity called *mast cells.*

The Capillary Bed and the Innate Immune System

Since the matrix is the oldest "organ system" in multicellular life-forms, it possesses only the more ancient or innate immune system and not the adaptive immune system that developed in higher animals. The innate pathway is found in all multicellular organisms and is the only immune system for plants, fungi, and insects. The adaptive immune system develops antigens or antidotes that respond to each invader and is able to retain a memory of the molecular configuration of offending substances and microbes so that it immediately recognizes them when they reappear and more quickly responds with antibodies and cytotoxins directed against them. This is the principle behind vaccination—exposure of the adaptive immune system to proteins so that it can form antidotes.

The innate immune system flashes into action when the perimeter has been breached and something enters the interior, whether it be a toxin, microbe, or thermic upset. At the front line of this internal defensive barrier are the pattern-recognition receptors, which are hardwired into both immune and, in lesser numbers, nonimmune cells. Pattern-recognition receptors will initiate the signaling that activates mast cells, one of the most primitive but still important and sophisticated immune cells, as well as neutrophils and macrophages. They begin by releasing antimicrobial agents and cytokines that signal additional responses. Mast cells are found in the connective tissue and congregated around the capillary bed and the lymphatics, under the skin and mucosa—especially of the lungs and intestines—or anywhere the perimeter is exposed to the exterior environment. Other immune cells are circulating in the blood, interstitial fluids, and lymph. Signals from the mast cells recruit neutrophils and monocytes that phagocytize (eat) microbes and toxins.

Mast cells are some of the most ancient immune cells. Responding to both pattern-recognition receptors and independent methods of activation, they quickly release *granules* containing histamine, heparin/heparan sulfate, and cytokines. The histamine dilates the blood vessels to allow phagocytizing neutrophils and macrophages to flow out of the capillaries and into the matrix. This causes the characteristic symptoms of inflammation (heat, redness, swelling, pain). The heparin/heparan sulfate undertakes numerous functions involving both immunity and normal functions of life in the matrix. The innate immune response marks the invading bacteria and substances for the arriving immune cells to phagocytize and destroy. The cytokines signal proteins circulating in the blood that activate the *complement cascade* that initiates an immune response that is complementary to and supplements the initial reaction by the mast cells, neutrophils, and macrophages. The immune response stimulates the macrophages to clear foreign and damaged wreckage from the area, maintains the inflammatory response, activates arriving immune cells, and initiates the *membrane attack complex,* which kills invading cells. It also promotes the removal of dead cells. Over thirty proteins compose the complement system, including proteins in the blood serum and cell membranes receptors. This accounts for about 10 percent of the proteinaceous globulin circulating in the bloodstream.

Mast cells act as a "major sensory arm of the innate immune system" that is sensitive to the appearance of pathogens and substances. In addition, these "sentinels" act as "regulatory cells" operating throughout the organism during an acute inflammatory reaction. "There is growing evidence that mast cells are key regulatory cells capable of coordinating and integrating many branches of the innate immune system." They even play a regulatory role in "immune contraction," which diminishes inflammatory responses so that the body may continue into granulation, and they continue a regulatory function all the way into the remolding phase (St. John and Abraham 2013, 4459–60).

When mast cell granules were introduced with vaccines, they caused an enhanced antigen-specific immune reaction (St. John and Abraham 2013, 4462). This shows that mast cells, though part of the innate immune system, stimulate the adaptive immune system, the source of the antigen-specific reaction. It also shows the vulnerability of different organisms to vaccines: some of them having too few mast cells and others too many.

When the mast cells overreact, we tend to get symptoms like allergic reactions, anaphylaxis, puffy red spots, and sudden redness. Characteristic remedies include Wild Cherry Bark, Rose Hips, Peach Leaf, Hawthorn, Linden flower, and homeopathic Apis mellifica (Honey bee—like treats like). Chronic mast cell overreaction is called mast cell activation syndrome (MCAS).

The innate immune system presents antigens or protein fragments for recognition to the adaptive immune system. The adaptive system reacts with specific antidotes to the offending antigens. These antidotes can include both a cell-mediated immune response by T cells and a humoral immune response, in the matrix, by B cells. They not only kill pathogens directly but also secrete antibodies that enhance the immune response, disrupting the infection.

The Capillary Bed, the Microbiome, and the Matrix

I made quite a point about the boundaries of the matrix being the capillary bed, the cell membrane, and the lymphatic capillary. Now I have to breach those boundaries. It turns out that the bacteria on the outside of the capillary bed have an influence on the matrix, and vice versa.

The original definition of the microbiome, in 1984, included the cells and the polymers associated with them (Elsen 2015). The technical name for the cells themselves is *microbiota*. There was tremendous wisdom in the original definition that was lost in subsequent sloppy thinking that changed the definition of the microbiome to the cells, solely. Just as the polymers in the ECM around the cells inside the organism control the matrix cells, the polymers used by the microbiota to construct and maintain their microbiome environment are also regulatory.

The microbiota are controlled by their environment, including molecules entering the organism from without, molecules generated by the microbiota, and those generated by the host organism. The microbiome communicates with the matrix via protein signals and substances that cross back and forth over the epithelial membrane. The mucin secreted by epithelial cells of the mucosa, which provides the environment for most of the microbiome, is developed out of serum and GAGs derived from the matrix. One of the primary paths of communication is through the immune system, with its protein-coded triggers and signals. These signals help to develop autoimmunity in the host. Changes in the ECM fibers, including collagen and fibronectin, occur as a result of changes in the microbiome (Sofat et al. 2015).

THE DETAILS OF "MIX"

The immune system of the interior of the matrix is simple because we are dealing with a method developed in the first multicellular organisms: the macrophage-fibroblast system. Macrophages consume microbes, allergens, broken-down cell parts, waste produces, and debris, while fibroblasts construct replacement parts to repair the damage that has occurred in the matrix and immune cells to replace those lost in the defensive battles inside the matrix. Both are present from the first stirrings of immune activity in the mast cells and inflammatory processes at the edge of the matrix, to the cells within, and to the lymphatic drainage out of the ECM—so they are centered in the mix department of the in-mix-out formula.

How does the matrix rebuild itself after a long, drawn out—or even a short—immune response to an external factor? Pischinger determined that the white blood cells (leukocytes) in the bloodstream, produced in the bone marrow and lymph nodes, are constantly breaking down; fragments flood into the matrix, where they are further broken down and actually act as an important food source for the cells of the matrix. The rate of manufacture and breakdown of the leukocytes is astonishing. There are an estimated 24 billion leukocytes in the body at any given time. Since they are manufactured at an estimated rate of 144 billion a day, in order for the number 24 billion to remain constant, 120 billion leukocytes need to be broken down during the same time period, or "1.2 million per second" (Pischinger 1991, 34). The process of leukocyte breakdown is constant and therefore a "non-specific process" (Pischinger 1991, 39).

This self-sacrificing aspect of the body's immune system helps feed and reboot the organism, nutritively. It is particularly helpful in the recovery stage after disease, when massive amounts of broken-down leukocytes are present. This makes leukocyte breakdown a part of the general adaptation syndrome described under homeostasis.

The GRS allows the passage of material favorable to life through the polymer sieve. Food gets to the cell membranes, where it is taken up by receptors that are keyed to each constituent arriving there: lipids, proteins, carbs, water, electrolytes, and others. The keyholes open and close due to chemical mediation (triggered by GRS signals) rather than pressure exerted against the cell by the matrix. The cells exert an outward pressure against the matrix in order to protect themselves against the passive pickup of materials and serum they don't need. The GRS signals interact with the cell membrane all the way to the nucleus of the cell.

The GRS also works on the basis of in-mix-out. Materials entering the matrix trigger electrical potential charges on the polymers of the

ECM, sending signals to the cells throughout the matrix, at the same time receiving signals from the cells about cell needs. These signals regulate the available mix for the cells. Waste materials do not carry an electrical charge, so they drift like abandoned ships until they are swept away into the Bermuda Triangle of the lymphatic system.

The life-supporting materials diffuse through the polymer sieve and immune mechanisms to get to the cell membranes. There, they are taken up by receptors that are keyed to each constituent—lipids, proteins, carbs, water, electrolytes, and others. The keyholes open and close due to chemical reactions rather than pressure, unlike the diffusion from the capillary bed into the matrix. In fact, the cells exert an outward pressure against the matrix that protects them against the passive pickup of materials and serum they don't want. These active uptake mechanisms are controlled by changes in electrical potential levels on the matrix polymers, influencing the electrical potential on the cell membrane. These chemical reactions are controlled by sodium and potassium ions that regulate the uptake and elimination of water in the cells and calcium ions that regulate the uptake of material.

High sodium and calcium levels can cause overfilling of the cells with water and other substances, resulting in a bloated matrix. This slows down the influx from the capillary bed, leading to a backup inside the capillaries and a backup of pressure along the vasculature, creating high blood pressure and an unhealthy back-pressure against the heart. This particular kind of blood pressure is controlled in biomedicine primarily by the use of calcium channel blockers. Sodium consumption is also limited, but the evidence for this is much more debatable. In fact, the most recent data suggests that moderate salt consumption is healthier than low consumption (Newman 2017). The race to blame salt, fats, and various proteins for high blood pressure now looks like a decades-long conspiracy for sugar producers to take the spotlight off the truly unhealthy food. We complementary and alternative medicine practitioners, being unruly and contrary to the medical establishment, have long held this position.

The electrical potential on the cell membrane is a product of energy production in the mitochondria inside the cell. They produce energy that is shipped via the ADP/ATP cycle to the cell membrane, which acts as a storage battery for the energy. Like any true battery, there has to be a negative pole and a positive pole. In this case, the former is on the inside of the cell membrane, while the latter is on the outside. That means that all living cells in the body have a positive external charge; this makes them mildly repellant to one another so that they don't aggregate and adhere together, although it makes them stick together once they have conjoined. If the generation and storage of energy is low, the cell membrane will have a low charge, resulting in congestion and adherence, trapping and blocking fluids in the matrix. Since the electrical potential on the cell membrane represents the energy reserve that keeps the cell healthy and prospering in its activities, a low charge is going to correlate with ill health (Moore 1989).

The glycocalyx surrounding the cell membrane is composed of polymers like those in the matrix, and both are charged negatively. The liquid-crystalline gel within which the polymers sit is negatively charged. Therefore, the matrix as a whole has a negative electrical potential charge, and because of this, it exerts a lesser pressure against the positively charged capillary bed and cell membranes. Receiving permission from the GRS, waste material from the greater circulation may move into the matrix. This includes blood proteins that creep in from the capillary bed (especially if there is an injury or inflammation), broken-down cells and cell parts from the blood, unused food, waste from cellular metabolism, dead (and living) bacteria, and viruses. If, for some reason, the cells cannot pick up all the food and material entering the matrix—perhaps because of sodium and calcium imbalances, among other things—then "food" will become a "waste product," further cluttering up the matrix.

Sodium ions control the uptake of water into the cells, while potassium ions are involved with the elimination of water and calcium ions with the uptake of solids. This is why sodium is diuretic (leading water out through the kidneys), potassium is lost through too much urination, and calcium channel blockers are used to prevent calcium from hardening up cell membranes and creating high blood pressure. This condition is also blamed on high sodium levels in the matrix and cells, causing fullness and back pressure against the capillary bed. Lack of potassium to balance the sodium also causes high blood pressure.

The electrical potential on the cell membrane is greater than that on the matrix polymers. As we have seen, this is a product of energy production in the mitochondria inside the cell. If the generation and storage of energy is low, the cell membrane will have a low charge, resulting in the clumping of cells together, since there is less repulsion between the positively charged cell membranes. Also, there is probably a pathological change in the electrical potential charge, which is negative. All of this results in congestion, blockage, and stoppage of fluid movement in the matrix. This causes clutter in the matrix and encourages bacterial feeding or toxin buildup.

Another molecule associated with the movement of water and waste toward the lymphatic outlets in cell salt teaching is sodium sulfate (homeopathic Natrum sulphuricum). This is a purgative (Glauber's salts) when used in large amounts. Homeopathic provings and clinical experience show that it moves water and water-borne contents. According to the cell salt doctors, it removes the debris from around the cells to the outlets (lymphatic capillaries) for removal. Sulphate is an extraordinary potent anion. As the major constituent of sulfation factor, it combines with protein sugars to form GAGs and PGs. It may be that some of the sulfates in the matrix polymers combine with the sodium congregating around them to form sodium sulphate, and there, in the depths of the matrix, this ion facilitates the removal of polymer debris.

"Bad Blood" or Waste in the Matrix

Pischinger (1991) calls the waste product in the matrix "slag." This is what a Western herbalist would call "bad blood," "impure blood," or "toxins in the blood." From Hippocrates to Culpeper, it would have been called "humors in the blood."

This very old and important concept holds that impurities or toxins build up in the blood that need to be removed by blood purifiers or alterative herbs. This folk medicine concept is not as outlandish as it sounds. These toxins are not actually in the blood, which is too highly controlled within strict parameters to tolerate this kind of thing. Instead, they collect in the matrix.

To my knowledge, the identification of "bad blood" with the matrix, rather than the blood itself, was first suggested by herbalist Paul Bergner.

> The "blood" of bad blood is not really the blood at all, but the extracellular fluid that bathes the cells. The blood itself only comprises about five percent of the fluids in the body, while the extracellular fluid makes up about twenty percent. The rest of the body's liquid lies within the cells. The extracellular fluid accumulates the metabolic wastes of all the cells, the waste byproducts of infection and inflammation, and toxic byproducts of poor digestion. When an infection spreads, it does so through this medium. With an overload of toxic substances in the extracellular fluid, any number of diseases can arise. The extracellular fluid then resembles Lake Erie more than it does the pristine lake in your favorite wilderness area. This polluted state of the extracellular fluid is, in my opinion, the best definition of "bad blood." (Bergner 1997)

This is certainly the correct identification of the physiological basis of "bad blood." It adds alteratives to the list of herbal medicines that operate on the matrix and its cellular inhabitants.

❧ Symptoms of "Bad Blood"

Traditionally, the usual symptoms of "bad blood" are seen in the skin, particularly as acne, eczema, or rashes of some kind. These are attributed to lack of elimination of "toxins" through the skin, kidneys, or colon, lack of good metabolism of waste products in the liver and cells, lack of good lymphatic drainage, or all three. There may also be hypothyroidism, causing a lower level of catabolism; in fact, the old name for hypothyroidism was "bad blood" (Barnes and Galton 1976). This was why iodine and seaweed were counted among the alteratives. In addition, laxatives are used to flush out the system.

The single most characteristic symptom of "bad blood," as I mentioned before, is a reddish tongue coated with a thick, adhesive, greasy, yellow coating. This indicates a general inflammatory condition of the body (red tongue) with a buildup of oils that are not being eliminated (yellow, sticky, greasy coating) (Clymer 1963). It is also seen in chronic smokers. Feeling hungover very easily in the morning, after a large meal, or after eating is also highly characteristic. Constipation is more typical, but diarrhea is not impossible.

The remedies for the mix phase are the alteratives, laxatives, the mucilages, and a stray bunch of herbs that we could call "restoratives," like Gotu Kola, Opuntia, and Comfrey. We are still learning about how to repair the matrix.

THE DETAILS OF "OUT"

Neither the matrix nor the lymphatics possess their own dedicated pump. The movement of water in and out of the matrix is therefore largely overseen by the pressure gradient between the capillary bed, the matrix, the cell, and the lymphatic capillaries. Sodium actively moves water into the cells, while potassium assists water movement out of the cells.

The pressure in the matrix, though lower than that in the capillary bed or the cell, is higher than what we find in the lymphatic capillaries, so matrix serum containing waste presses up against and into flaps in the lymphatic capillaries, which are only one epithelial layer thick in the matrix. Through the lymphatics, the waste and serum drains off into the lymphatic system, conveying this lymph to the circulation, which finally brings it to the liver and kidneys for processing and elimination.

The lymphatics are the major outlet in the in-mix-out formula, but they are assisted by the venules—the distal end of the capillary bed—which take the CO_2 and H_2O remnants of cellular metabolism. The venules rely on the fall in pressure after the capillary bed has emptied the serum and its contents into the matrix. The pressure in the capillary bed falls so that wastewater, carbon dioxide, ions, and very small particles are pushed back into the venules, which move these wastes toward the lungs for expulsion.

One of the waste products of cell metabolism is water. This will not be in the liquid-crystalline form (H_3O+/H_2O_2-), but will be plain, ordinary H_2O. This, as we have seen, is not the kind of water used in a living organism. This wastewater, with carbon dioxide and small particles, is pushed back into the venules, which have low pressure due to all the serum and blood contents that were extruded into the matrix from the arterial end of the capillaries. The CO_2 and H_2O are moved to the lungs for elimination: the vapor of our breath is the wastewater of cellular metabolism.

As we have seen, the polymers in the matrix are arranged like graceful feathers or wings that fold up and unfold due to the amount of water fluffing them up. They are constantly being generated by the fibroblasts to replace any polymers that break down. However, they have their weak structural points, and they are always getting torn and ragged-edged. There has to be a mechanism in the body for combing through these proteoglycans and breaking off the weak bits. This may be a function of the macrophages, responsible for waste removal, but the cell salt theory gives a different explanation: the work of trimming old structural material away is undertaken by a small amount of free silicon circulating in the waters of the body.

Silicon is the sharpest of all bio-active elements; even in its smallest natural form (Si_2), it is sharp. In the mineral kingdom around us, silicon accounts for sharpness: flint is pure silicon and glass is an aluminosilicate. According to the cell salt theory, silicon is seen as the "homeopathic scalpel" that trims what we would now call the matrix polymers. Thus, the silicon molecules present in the matrix enter into and act on the proteoglycan polymers, collagens, cartilage, sinews, and bones. While this is going on, a certain amount of silicon precipitates out of solution and shows up as a 1 percent content level in bones and connective tissue. The amount of silicon in solution is very small at any given moment, but it is crucial (according to this theory) in the free flow of the interstitial fluids, and perhaps even for the electrical potential charge on healthy polymers.

The constant "pruning" of bits and pieces of matrix polymer that are losing integrity opens up the ECM so that the serum flow through the tissues is less hindered; this in turn allows for a slight outward diffusion of fluid and heat through the body, toward the periphery. By keeping the diffusion of fluids and heat gently toward the surface, silicon has a faint but important externalizing, cleansing effect. Herbs that are high in silicon probably assist in this movement. One of them would be Horsetail (*Equisetum arvense, E. hyemale*) and another would probably be Teasel (*Dipsacus* spp.)

Leaving Silicon aside, the major remedies for the out aspect of the matrix would be the lymphatic herbs, particularly Cleavers, Red Root, Calendula, Violet Leaf, Red Clover, Poke Root (small dose), Scrophularia, Ocotillo *(Fouquieria splendens),* and Echinacea. Gravel Root opens up the lymphatic capillaries, although it is not considered a lymphatic remedy. Echinacea is the only strong stimulant in the bunch so it can be used to potentiate a lymphatic formula.

Conclusion

I could never understand physiology or pathophysiology on the molecular level until I read about the matrix—then it began to make sense. As an intuitive, I needed to understand the greater whole, the context within which physiology operated. It was impossible for me to appreciate literature that happily discussed the parts without offering a view of the whole. Something seemed intrinsically, deeply, even disturbingly wrong with a system that could not explain context.

I did not expect to ever run across an explanation for holism in the hard science, but Alfred Pischinger provided that foundation. If I have lauded him to the skies when so many other authors ignore him, that is my excuse. He doesn't get much credit, by the way: all the papers on the ECM I read, except those by Harmut Heine, did not mention him. Conventional medicine and science not only wanted to forget that the basic premise of holism had replaced the basic tenet of reductionism—the cell theory—but it wanted to forget the medical doctor who had painstakingly put together the pieces to form the whole.

I did not write this book for a conventional audience. Because I have been only modestly trained in reading papers, evaluating evidence, and presenting scientific data, I anticipate some arguments against my presentation, but there is one area where I challenge science, and this is perspective. Just as perspective uncovers the difference between an artist who is a professional and one that is an amateur, so must it operate in the theater of our knowledge. And so far, perspective has been assumed and not examined as a scientific subject.

It is for intuitives and adherents of holistic medicine, like myself, that I write. We need to understand, not only that our "theory" (as Pischinger called it) is justified, but also how it changes our perspective. Not only do we need to know that this premise is explained by hard science, we need to know how to exploit that knowledge with appropriate treatment modalities. Finally, as I have said, nobody is going to write our holistic books unless we do it ourselves.

Appendix

Homeostasis: Balance in the Matrix

The fixity of the milieu supposes a perfection of the organism such that the external variations are at each instant compensated for and equilibrated. . . . All of the vital mechanisms, however varied they may be, have always one goal, to maintain the uniformity of the conditions of life in the internal environment. . . . The stability of the internal environment is the condition for the free and independent life.

CLAUDE BERNARD

(QUOTED IN GROSS 1998, 383)

Now we will move on to an overview of the basic processes and patterns that regulate the natural flux of the extracellular matrix. This includes (1) terminology describing balance, stress, and response in the organism (2) patterns of imbalance, and (3) different types of reactions to medicinal substances. These concepts were difficult for me to grasp, they are difficult to explain, and, because of this, I feel this chapter may be awkwardly written at times. So I want to apologize to you at the outset. There is also the problem that Cannon and Selye, who developed our understanding of homeostasis, stress, and adaptation, worked long before many of the discoveries in this book. Therefore, their discussion is limited to the neuroendocrine system.

197

HOMEOSTASIS

An American doctor, Walter Cannon (1871–1945), studied in Paris and particularly esteemed Claude Bernard, whose milieu intérieur lead inevitably to Cannon's concept of *homeostasis*. This term describes the ongoing self-regulation of the organism in a steady state. The word *homeostasis* conveys the idea that the body always seeks to return to a like (*homeo*) state (*stasis*).

> The coordinated physiological reactions which maintain most of the steady states in the body are so complex, and are so peculiar to the living organism, that [I have] suggested . . . that a specific designation for these states be employed—homeostasis. (Cannon 1929, 400)

Homeostasis was not just a concept, however. Cannon also was trying to explain the operation of the adrenal medulla and the hormones associated with it: adrenaline (epinephrine) and noradrenaline (norepinephrine). He coined the phrase "fight-or-flight" to explain the action of these hormones.

The function of the adrenal medulla was thus understood, but not that of the adrenal cortex. Working over the next few years, Hans Selye (1907–1982) applied the idea of homeostasis to explain the action of the adrenal cortex and its hormones. Some of these act on the inflammatory response, either to enhance or suppress it. Cannon and Selye considered the chief function of the adrenals to be adaptation to stress. Cannon introduced these terms but Selye popularized them, and they are, in fact, associated with his name much more so than with Cannon's. The activities of the adrenals are complex and we are only looking at a part of their function here.

The next big piece of biological knowledge that the milieu intérieur concept helped bring into place was the concept of *cybernetics,* which was developed by Norbert Wiener (1894–1964). This idea is now broadly applied to any communication network that contains a feedback loop. Feedback reinforces regulatory signals that maintain the status quo in the system using the loop. Although originally applied to biological organisms and nonliving machines, the term *cybernetics* is now applied to human society and communication between completely different life-forms or between life-forms and inanimate systems. In the biological realm, it is used, for instance, to describe communication between different plants, bacteria, fungi, and soils that, altogether, produce an environmental biome. It is also used to describe communication between the bacterial biome in the gut and the animal organism.

When Alfred Pischinger mapped out, defined, and explained the GRS, at last the basic constituents and functions of the milieu intérieur were understood. The GRS is, of course, a cybernetic system of self-regulation for the matrix and the cells.

The grand implications of all of these advances in science are known to modern biomedicine, but they are not used in therapy. Instead, biomedicine circumvents homeostasis and the GRS by directing powerful molecules (drugs) to the receptor sites in cell membranes, circumventing cybernetic self-regulation, weakening the GRS, and leading to new symptoms, problems, diseases, and, ultimately, unnecessary fatalities. Similar shortsightedness rules in modern agriculture, which destroys the plant biome by growing genetically engineered monocrops using herbicides and pesticides that kill virtually everything but the crop—including the biome. Industry, using these crops, has manufactured foods that irritate the biome in the gut and therefore may disrupt important communication systems. The crudeness and destructiveness of these practices will be looked on in the future—if pharmaceutical and pesticide practices do not destroy us first (a real possibility)—as far more damaging than medieval medicine. Meanwhile, we of the alternative wing, who set homeostasis as our goal and treat the organism as a whole using gentle remedies, are looked on as ignorant pseudoscientists. Holistic medicine is the only approach based on the modern scientific principles of homeostasis, stress, cybernetics, holistic treatment, and genuine cure via a return to self-maintenance in the organism.

ALLOSTASIS

More recently, in 1988, the concept of *allostasis* was introduced by Peter Sterling and Joseph Eyer to describe a different avenue for restoration to homeostasis. Whereas homeostasis is looked on as a gentle fluctuation that carries organic processes back and forth in response to mild environmental changes, allostasis describes a state in which the organism has to deal with stresses that are temporarily or permanently overwhelming. A healthy organism carries the extra stress for a while—this is called the *allostatic load*—until it can rally its forces and return the body to the more or less original homeostatic balance. This would describe a fever, in which the body heats up, cytokines are generated, the immune system responds, and there is a period of disease followed by resolution. If there is no healthy resolution, the organism continues in allostasis.

Both homestasis and allostasis are looked on as responses that return the organism to balance. The term *allostasis* derives from the Greek *allo* (alien, foreign, different from, variation), so *allostasis* means "remaining stable in variation," that is, the "new norm."

RHEOSTASIS

The term *rheostasis* is now also used to account for the fact that animals change levels of steady state to deal with different kinds of stress and biological need. For instance, the body sets the thermostat higher to produce a fever, to accelerate metabolism and eliminate waste products, then returns to "normal." Metabolism can be different in the winter from the summer—one reason Minnesotans gain weight in the winter and lose it (hopefully) in the summer.

STRESS AND ADAPTATION

The GRS was not known at the time of Cannon and Selye. Therefore, they defined stress and adaptation in terms of the sympathetic and parasympathetic branches of the autonomic nervous system (ANS), which, with the endocrine system, regulates the major organs and functions.

We now know that the major regulatory systems of the body include the GRS as well as the endocrine and nervous systems, and that the latter two pass hormones and neurotransmitters through the matrix as part of a cybernetic loop. Hormones pass through the matrix to get from the producing cell to the receptor cell, while neurotransmitters are dumped into the matrix at the nerve ending, travel through the ECFs to the lymph, the blood, and then the hypothalamus, the grand regulatory center of the neuroendocrine center, where they are analyzed by the hypothalamus. We also know, as some of our chapters show, that the GRS mediates defense and recovery on the tissue and cell levels. Therefore, it would be accurate to define homeostasis and allostasis in terms related to the GRS, in combination with the neuroendocrine system.

The ANS is the regulatory system that acts without conscious oversight through the unconscious functions of the body, such as heart rate, vascular control, blood distribution, digestion, respiratory rate, urination, sexual arousal, and pupillary response in the eyes. The sympathetic nervous system originates in and runs along the vertebra. It revs up to the fight-or-flight response level, but it also just simply keeps us alive and aware the rest of the time. As opposed to the sympathetic, the parasympathetic is responsible for rest, relaxation, digestion, and rebuilding. It arises in nerve plexi lying along the inner side of the spinal cord.

Stress

This term was introduced by Cannon to describe irritants in the physical or emotional environment that throw off homeostasis.

Although stress is usually used in a negative sense, it is technically divided into two subdivisions: *distress* (negative stress that overwhelms the defenses of the body through intensity, destructiveness, or length of time), and *eustress* (positive stress that is manageable, engages the resources of the organism, and leads to growth and enhanced competence). Modern research on mice, babies, children, and adults shows that stress, when brought to a healthy resolution, builds both mental and physical health by allowing the organism to adapt to new circumstances and become more resilient. The key is for the stress not to reach a level where it overwhelms our capacity to respond. When stress is so extreme that it cannot be brought to resolution, it is termed *trauma*.

It is interesting to think how some people thrive in extremely stressful situations but not in others, as if their system was set to be stimulated by high levels of stress. An example of this would be Oskar Schindler, the Czech-German industrialist who actively opposed the Nazi regime to save thousands of Jews, yet was a complete failure during peacetime. It was as if his charisma and strength were suited *only* to a condition of extreme and constant danger.

Although Cannon introduced the term *stress,* it was Selye who popularized the word, which today is ubiquitous in both professional and popular medicine. We now tend to use it in conversation to describe events and people that cause us psychological or nervous upset, but it equally applies to weather, food, microorganisms, and in fact anything at all that can upset our biological equilibrium. Recall that these factors are called stressors.

Selye was very pleased with the word *stress.* He was a native of central Europe, conversant in five European languages, and concluded that the English word *stress* was the only term in any of these languages that fulfilled the meaning that was needed to describe the intention he and Cannon had for this concept.

There are three basic pathways by which the organism can respond to stress, according to Cannon and Selye. All three are associated with the ANS. The sympathetic branch supports the fight-or-flight response, while the parasympathetic supports both the inflammatory response and its suppression. The sympathetic and the parasympathetic are mutually suppressive: we are either in one or the other. The adrenal cortex generates the pro-inflammatory response via what Selye termed mineralocorticoid hormones and the anti-inflammatory response via glucocorticoid hormones. In homeostasis, these oppose and balance each other. This means that we basically have a three-pronged response to stress.

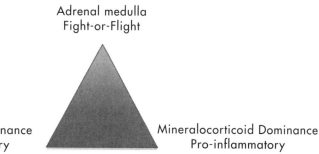

The three-pronged response to stress in humans.

ࣷ Stress Hormones

In response to acute stress, the sympathetic initiates a hormonal response starting in the adrenal medulla that raises the secretion of catecholamines (noradrenaline and adrenaline). This is called the *short-term stress response* or sympathomedullary (SAM) pathway because it involves the sympathetic nervous system and the adrenal medulla. This is characterized by an increase in heart rate, respiration, and blood sugar levels, so that the person or animal is ready to fight or flee.

Another pathway is responsible for the long-term stress response. The hypothalamus reads the changes in the blood sugar levels, sends a signal (coricotropin-releasing hormone or CRH) to the pituitary, which in turn sends a signal (adrenocorticotropic hormone, ACTH, or adrenocrtico-stimulating hormone, ACSH) to the adrenal cortex, which releases cortisol. Therefore, this is called the hypothalamo-pituitary-adrenal pathway (or HPA axis). Cortisol is the hormone that runs the long-term stress response. It raises blood sugar levels, increases the appetite, and reduces or controls the inflammatory response in the other corner of the adrenal cortex, diminishing mineralocorticoid secretion.

The third response to stress occurs through the last mentioned mechanism, the mineralocorticoid corner. The hypothalamus signals the pituitary, which signals the thyroid with thyroid-stimulating hormone (TSH). This turns up the heat in the body and favors the inflammatory response. The mineralocorticoid corner promotes increased diuresis (via aldosterone), increased liver, thyroid, and immune system (via androgens), and decreased cortisol output via dehydroepiandrosterone, popularly known as DHEA.

I was irritated by Selye's two terms, *glucocorticoid* and *mineralocorticoid,* because they seemed so abstruse and technical. However, he explains that the glucocorticoid hormone cortisol raises glucose levels, while the mineralocorticoid hormones raise the salt (mineral) level in the blood to produce a more lean, mean, fightin' machine. For popular consumption, Selye invented the terms type A and type B to describe people. Type A is mineralocorticoid-dominant, hotter, quicker to respond, more aggressive, and angry if thwarted, with an active thyroid, liver, and kidneys. Type B is more mellow, slow to anger and respond, thoughtful, but prone to weight gain—the Winnie the Pooh type. There should also be a third type, who is thin, nervous, and quick to respond in a nervous fashion, because they are dominated by the sympathomedullary (SAM) response.

When we look at the three corners of the stress response triangle, we see how long-term constitutional stress response mechanisms form our constitutional type. Using the three types from Ayurvedic medicine (vata, pitta, kapha), we have: thin, nervous, tense (vata or ectomorph);

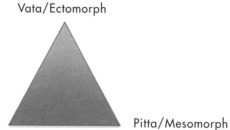

The constitutional types matched to the three corners
of the stress response triangle.

strong, muscular, active, hot (pitta or mesomorph); and slow, thick, meditative (kapha or endomorph).

Adaptation

The ability of the organism to respond to stress is called *adaptation*. This includes both the ability to return to homeostasis as well as the ability to establish a new equilibrium—temporary or permanent— that is not based on a return to homeostasis but one in which the organism keeps operating with unresolved stresses in place.

THREE DIFFERENT KINDS OF STRESS RESPONSE

It is not at all easy to understand the three stress pathways described on the preceding three pages, and I did so using my own terminology and images to attempt to bring order to the subject. Now I am going to represent the ideas according to how Cannon and Selye framed the terminology.

Fight-or-Flight (or Freeze)

The characteristic symptoms of the adrenaline reaction are perception of sudden danger, instantaneous increased awareness, blood to the brain and limbs, less to the viscera, increased heart rate and blood pressure, pale or flushed skin, lowered pain response, dilated pupils, anxiety, tension, or even trembling. Through constant use of the pathway, symptoms can become chronic.

General Adaptation Syndrome

Selye found that all stressors can cause either a *nonspecific, general reaction* or a *specific, local reaction*. He called these the general adaptation syndrome (GAS) and the local adaptation syndrome (LAS). The former represents a general, all-body response caused by the domination of cortisol, which suppresses the inflammatory response of the mineralocorticoid corner of the adrenal cortex. This is characterized by three basic changes: enlargement of the adrenal cortex; shrinkage of the thymus, spleen, and lymphatic glands; and stimulation of the gastrointestinal tract. The LAS represents a local, articulated, and individualized immune response that is different for each different kind of stress. This is what medicine in all times and places, ancient and modern, has largely addressed. The general adaptation syndrome, is a completely different pathway that helps the organism adapt to stress and overcome it without undergoing the local immune response depending on the mineralocorticoids, which increase inflammation and detoxification. Selye envisioned the GAS response in three characteristic stages: *alarm, resistance,* and *exhaustion.*

The GAS was not consciously addressed by medicinal agents until 1948, when a Soviet scientist, Dr. Nikolai Lazarev, introduced the term *adaptogen.* The first agent so defined was *Eleutherococcus senticosis,* used by Siberian hunters to increase stamina and resistance to environmental stress while sojourning in the wilderness. In retrospect it was realized that many "tonic" herbs, especially the mushrooms used in traditional Chinese medicine, were adaptogenic, and now the category is well established.

Alarm Stage: After encountering a stressor, the body reacts with the fight-or-flight response, activating the sympathetic branch of the

ANS. The stress hormones cortisol and adrenaline are released into the bloodstream to meet the threat, danger, or attack. This mobilizes the body's resources. Cortisol moves from the short term adrenaline response to long term.

Resistance Stage: The parasympathetic mode of the ANS returns many physiological functions to normal levels while the body focuses resources against the stressor. Blood glucose levels remain high and cortisol and adrenaline continue to circulate at elevated levels, but the body remains on alert. However, it is able to function more easily to take care of the business of daily life. An increase in heart rate, blood pressure, and respiration remains.

Exhaustion Stage: If the stressor continues to burden the organism beyond its capacity, the resources of the organism are exhausted and it becomes susceptible to chronic illness.

If the stress finally lets up, the organism may be able to deal with the stress in a constructive manner, leading to a successful resolution. The relax, rest, and digest wing of the ANS is the parasympathetic nervous system. It works in concert with the sympathetic nervous system, and it uses and activates the release of the neurotransmitter acetylcholine. Its main function is to return the organism to homeostasis after stress. Acetylcholine opposes the catecholamines that favor fight or flight.

Selye's concept of the exhaustion stage seems to have led to the concept of "adrenal exhaustion," a widely used folk medicine term that is rejected by biomedicine. If we stick to Selye's concept, however, we see that it is a real condition.

The adrenaline response is inexhaustible because the body always needs to be able to mount a reaction to danger. However, the adrenocortical hormones are limited. The continuing release of adrenaline keeps the body in a constant sympathetic excess that suppresses the parasympathetic. These two pathways are mutually exclusive: when one is on, the other is off. Therefore, the body can't digest, rest, relax, and rebuild sufficiently, so the adrenal cortex which supports parasympathetic function is chronically undernourished. The adrenal cortex requires lipids. These are hard to digest and assimilate when the organism is in sympathetic overdrive, so it weakens and there is undersecretion of glucocorticoids and mineralocorticoids.

The misunderstanding has arisen that "exhaustion" refers to adrenaline, which cannot be exhausted. As Selye explains, it is the other resources of the body, dependent on the parasympathetic, that are exhausted. There is constant overstimulation and overreaction with a constant shortage of staying power.

Local Adaptation Syndrome

The specific local reactions association with this syndrome differentiate all conditions and diseases, introducing reactions specific to each stressor, resulting in the characteristic symptoms by which we recognize and name pathologies. These are also the symptoms for which we prescribe a drug or herb. Like the GAS, the LAS can also become exhausted; if it does, it may initiate general adaptation.

> The selective exhaustion of muscles, eyes, or inflamed tissue all represent final stages only in local adaptation syndromes (L.A.S.). Several of these may go on simultaneously in various parts of the body, and in proportion to their intensity and extent, they can activate the G.A.S.-mechanism. (Selye 1956, 65)

Exhaustion of the GAS leads to death. "Only when all of our adaptability is used up will irrevocable, general exhaustion and death take place" (Selye 1956, 66).

The catalog of stressors normally encountered in the course of a lifetime can be reduced to a somewhat short list.

> Prolonged exertion, noise, infection, exposure to cold and heat, shock, fatigue, decreased oxygen supply, pain, malnutrition,

radiation, obesity, anger, fear, old age, excitement, anxiety, pregnancy, injuries, drugs, disease, medical treatment, and surgery account for most of the stressors with which the physiologist is concerned. (Ramsey 1982, 34)

He left out the nasty ones: poverty, abuse, congenital weaknesses, wounds, accidents, and probably some more.

❧ Adaptive Energy as Innate Vitality

Adaptation represents the ability of the organism to oppose stress. Selye (1956, 66) characterized it as an "energy."

The term *adaptation energy* has been coined for that which is consumed during continued adaptive work, to indicate that it is something different from the caloric energy we receive from food; but this is only a name, and we still have no precise concept of what this energy might be. Further research along these lines would seem to hold great promise, since here we appear to touch upon the fundamentals of aging. (Selye 1956)

Selye's "adaptation energy" is similar to what we would call "constitutional strength" in popular speech. He saw it as innate inherited vitality which was strengthened by overcoming stresses during life.

It is as though, at birth, each individual inherited a certain amount of adaptation energy, the magnitude of which is determined by his genetic background, his parents. He can draw upon this capital thriftily for a long but monotonously uneventful existence, or he can spend it lavishly in the course of a stressful, intense, but perhaps more colorful and exciting life. In any case, there is just so much of it, and he must budget accordingly. (Selye 1956, 66)

In a particularly beautiful passage, Selye discusses the art of life, sounding almost like one of the old philosophers or alchemists discussing the "Great Work."

> The great art is to express our vitality through the particular channels and at the particular speed which nature foresaw for us. (Selye 1956, 269)

HIPPOCRATIC TREATMENT, OR GOOD NURSING TECHNIQUE

The GAS response teaches us to appreciate the logic of the ancient Hippocratic method, which emphasized very basic healing techniques. By removing stressors (such as food difficult to digest or metabolize) and promoting rest, sleep, and dream, patients generally got better, unless they were too far gone already—even then, they might live longer, in better comfort. These are, of course, the basics of home treatment and professional nursing down to the present. The attempt to remove environmental and food allergens is an important part of naturopathic and holistic treatment today. These methods are probably even more important today, when the general population in inundated by irritants and toxins, the natures of which are little known, or even if known, still used to perpetuate corporate profits or public convenience.

In dealing with the Hippocratic writings, we are not, of course, dealing with an individual, but with a group of people who saw themselves as members of the same school and who identified with the name Hippocrates. Thus, there are contradictory approaches and methods found within the Hippocratic writings. However, the themes considered most characteristic of the scientific impulse in Hippocrates revolve around simple methods of diet and hygiene. The basic method of treatment, according to this approach, was to promote rest and a bland, nourishing, but not—as we would say today—stressful diet.

Such methods, as Selye points out, are the timeless tools used by doctors, nurses, and laypeople to promote healing. He notes that these methods are nonspecific and are particularly well suited to the general adaptation response.

Selye did not deny that heroic treatments were also used in traditional medicine. He believed that there was a logic to these approaches as well. As he explained, a local disease associated with an LAS would be extinguished by a stressor that moved the disease from a local to a general expression, eliciting a healing response through the GAS. He himself had watched his father, a medical doctor, apply bloodletting, a widespread European medical technique used as late as the 1950s. He believed that this elicited a response that moved the disease from local to general adaptation, making basic nursing techniques applicable.

I don't want to drag the reader into arcane corners of alternative medicine but I can't think of any other literary opportunity I will ever have to discuss the following important point. The technique described by Selye in the last paragraph, initiating a general adaptation response, is exactly the opposite to the homeopathic approach, which seeks to initiate a specific reaction through the use of a specific medicinal agent (the local adaptation syndrome). This is also true of "specific medicine," a movement in herbalism based on the use of specific herbs associated with specific local actions—my favorite kind of herbalism.

Selye noticed that the Hippocratic physicians defined disease not only as *pathos* (suffering) but *ponos* (hardship, toil). He looked upon this as a tacit acknowledgment of the existence of stress. It takes work to remain in health, and this implies a force that is fighting against oneself continually, in health and in disease. Both alternative and conventional practitioners would agree that many people don't want to work to remain healthy.

In Hippocratic medicine, the energy in the organism that provides the capacity to heal is termed *physis*. This word simply means

"Nature," so it is Nature within the organism that resists hardship and promotes healing. *Physis,* therefore, is a lot like the concept of the vital force stripped down to the bare minimum: it is Nature within us that maintains our health, just as it is Nature that buoys up all of the life around us.

Because the GAS response encourages good home treatment and nursing, an excellent review of Selye's work appears on the website currentnursing.com, under the tab nursing theories.

INFLAMMATION, THE MOTHER OF ALL DISEASE

Another unifying concept is that of inflammation. The process of oxidation is the basis of life and death. We have already discussed these subjects in past chapters; at this juncture we are going to look at different pathways that lead to or result from inflammation. In other words, we are going to look at basic processes and patterns of disease origination. These are essentially patterns of local adaptation. Patterns are one of the most important foundations for holistic medicine.

The Six Tissue States

I frequently speak or write of the six tissue states, a system of description of pathophysiology I revived from nineteenth-century medicine (particularly from Thurston 1900). The terminology is still used in biomedicine today, but the difference is that today the tissue states are used to describe pathology, whereas in nineteenth-century medicine (allopathic, homeopathic, physiomedical, eclectic), they were also used as a basis for prescription and the practice of medicine.

Excitation or Irritation: This represents an overreaction of the inflammatory response or, as we would say today, an autoimmune excess condition. Circulation, nervous activity, heat, redness, etc., are all exaggerated.

This is the state that needs coolants or refrigerants, sedatives, and antioxidants. There are three degrees of heat in Greek medicine, represented by three pulses: superficial (immune overreactivity), rapidity (inflammation, fever), and quick (no space between the beats, mental restlessness, insomnia, mania, etc.—in fact, exaggerated fight-or-flight).

Depression: The opposite side of the pole from excitation is depression, which represents a lack of reactivity to stress. There may be a lack of circulation to the extremities, enervation, or immune response. The characteristic symptoms are low body temperature, pallor of the surface or dark complexion (due to lack of circulation), inactive diaphoresis, and other functional weaknesses. This is the state that responds to stimulants (usually spices) and diffusives (remedies that tingle). In Greek medicine, the three degrees of cold are associated with the rare pulse (long spaces between the beats, athletic tone), slow pulse (lack of energy), and low pulse (poor circulation and innervation). Inflammation results from deteriorating tissue (no circulation or innervation) and is usually associated with bacteria feeding off these conditions. Bacteria, through the release of endotoxins, depress tissue function.

Tension or Constriction: When the nerves can't relax, a state of tension, either psychological or physical, results. Tension or tightness in nerves and circulation causes alternating congestion or drying of tissues that can result in inflammation, so the characteristic symptoms are usually chills, chills alternating with heat, diarrhea alternating with constipation, alternating and sudden onset of symptoms, and a tense or tight pulse. The remedies here are acrid (the taste of bile in the back of the throat), from Valerian to the DMT hallucinogens.

Relaxation: Here the tissues lack tone, starting with the pores, so that the initial symptoms are those of fluid loss. This is followed by loose, saggy, boggy tissue, and eventually prolapse. The passage of fluids over the tissues from open pores initially causes cooling, but tissues damp for a long time result in rotting and inflammation. The tongue is damp, so its coating (if at all) is white. The remedies in Western herbalism are the astringents; in Chinese herbalism, this condition is called "yang deficiency" and the usual remedies are "yang tonics" that gently warm; in Western astrological medicine, the gentle warming herbs are called "solar remedies."

Atrophy: First there is drying out from lack of the two "yin" substances: water and/or oil. Since nutrition occurs via the waterways of the body (blood, lymph, interstitial fluids, CSF), darkness next causes atrophy. Lack of oils also causes atrophy. The tongue and skin are usually dry in the first degree, thin in the second, and creviced in the third. This shows the progression from dryness to atrophy to damage. The pulse is usually narrow on one side and tense on the other. Remedies are moistening and nutritive.

The issue of the aging and stiffening of the components of the matrix comes up for consideration primarily under this tissue state. As tissue ages, proteins that form junctions between fibers decrease, compromising all the great things the fibers have been upholding for the organism, reducing pliability, strength, and softness, and opening gaps between epithelial cells lining the mucosa and skin so that tissues are both more permeable and less flexible. The basement membrane thins, fibroblasts stop reproducing, and cells become resistant to apoptosis. These senescent changes encourage pathological destruction (inflammation, bacterial infection) instead of natural breakdown; they also promote cancer. The combination of inflammation and changed constituents encourages the destruction of the integrity of the elastin network and basement membrane. At the same time that the appropriate cross-linkage is deteriorating, inappropriate collagen fibers conjoin tissues, making structures weaker, less elastic, and more rigid. These processes are encouraged by oxidation and exposure to sunlight.

Stagnation or Torpor: There are two types of dampness: flowing and stagnation. Relaxation of the tissues (described above) results in the loss of fluids because the relaxed pores and sphincters can't hold on to the fluids. This was described above under "Relaxation." This second type of dampness results in fluid buildup because there is a lack of channels or open pores to pass through. Water is cooling and flowing, and that is what is lost in the relaxed tissue state, but in stagnation or torpor, there seems to be an excess of unmetabolized oils, and these cause blockage and inflammation. This is shown by a red tongue body (inflammation) covered with a with a thick, adhesive, sticky, yellow coating (retained lipids). This is the classic indication for the use of alteratives, according to Dr. R. Swinburne Clymer (1878–1966), one of the last physiomedical physicians. In addition, the skin may be too oily or too dry, and skin eruptions are characteristic. It is believe that there is retention of toxins or metabolites with poor elimination via the skin, kidneys, colon, or lungs, so this supports inflammation.

We can see that these tissue states can be referred easily to the matrix, where there may be an excess or deficiency of immune reaction, which occurs in the capillary bed and areas rich in nerves. Or there may be too much or too little fluid in the matrix. Tension will only indirectly influence the matrix.

The tissue states also direct our eye to the question of treatment strategy. There are many different ways to conceptualize the use of medicinal substances.

PRINCIPLES OF MEDICINAL ACTION

The basis for establishing the action of a drug on the body is defined as the "structure/function claim" in modern pharmacology and medicine. The molecular structure of the drug reacts on the molecular structure of the target tissue in a precise way that changes the function of the tissue. The same model is applied in biomedicine to the herb. This approach requires the herb to be given in large enough doses to have a mechanical reaction. The problem with this approach was pointed out by Pischinger: it suppresses the innate regulatory systems of the body. While suppressing local symptoms, it weakens the overall integrity and self-governance of the body. When seen in this light, modern pharmacological medicine looks as primitive as medieval medicine.

When I was a young herbalist in the early eighties, working in the herb shop, I was taught to avoid using the term *"cure."* The only time one can use this term is in recounting a past case history in which a person was cured. After a while, I noticed that the medical doctors also avoided using this term and also that the phrase "health maintenance" became a byword at this time. In other words, the goal of medicine was no longer to cure but to maintain health. This is good in the preventive sense, but there is a darker inference: pay us to maintain your health, rather than relying on Nature *(physis)* and hard work *(ponos)*.

The basis of modern therapy is the randomized, double-blind, controlled drug trial (RCT). It involves plotting out the results on a graph. The normal positive reactions form a bulge or high curve on the graph, while the people who under- or overreacted to the therapy fall on either side, off the curve. Because it looks like a bell, the curve is known as a "bell curve." It doesn't actually take much of a curve to get a drug approved; this explains the large quantity of modern drugs that either don't cause a reaction or cause an overreaction.

I once wrote that modern medicine does not treat the individual but the "bulge on the Bell curve." My late friend Clara Niiska, a Native American anthropology Ph.D. student at the University of Minnesota, laughed until tears ran down her cheeks. "As in Georg Friedrich Bell," she intoned, imitating a serious white scientist. "Inventor of the Bell curve." My mistake was unintentional, but Clara saw this as a wonderful parody of the self-important science of the dominant culture. Another Native comic, Will Rogers, once commented that "back in the old days, in the Indian Territories, they used to just cure a person. Nowadays they send you from one specialist to another" (author's paraphrase).

Is there no basis for the curative art? Why is it that every traditional society, including our own, has always talked about "cure"? I notice that even today, laypeople talk about it and assume that medicine is on the same track. No, the basic supposition of modern biomedicine is that Nature cannot take care of herself. Once broken, there is no way to return her to health.

Pharmacology and the Immune System

The structure/function orientation to drug therapy is based on a mechanical effect. This forces the organism to act in a new way that overrides the GRS and self-maintenance by the organism. It is therefore not curative at all. It artificially maintains the organism in an altered, unnatural state—remember health maintenance?

The medical industry does not look for cure because there is no pay-off in cure. Maintenance is profitable. Big Pharma can't afford to spend nearly a billion dollars to introduce a drug that is curative. This has led to the idea that broken Nature cannot cure herself, that there is no cure. There is nothing scientific about this; it is another example of lack of perspective.

There is a molecular basis for the curative art, and the more progressive pharmacologists and physicians have been studying this phenomenon for a long time. This research involves the immune system, the natural self-healing faculty within the body.

Research undertaken by A. Friedman and H. L. Weiner in 1994 demonstrated that antigens acted through the bystander reaction mechanism of the immune system to create inflammation (Friedman and Weiner 1994). In 1996, Weiner and F. Meyer published a comprehensive overview of the literature of low-dose antigen reactions in the *Annals of the New York Academy of Sciences* (Weiner and Meyer 1996). In 1998, Hartmut Heine and Dr. Manfred Schmolz published an article titled "Induction of the Immunological Bystander Reaction by Plant Extracts" in *Biomedical Therapy* (Heine and Schmolz 1998).

The bystander reaction mechanism is an immune pathway that relies on macrophages to consume foreign material, toxins, and bacteria. It triggers a T cell reaction that promotes production of the messenger substance TGF-β. This cytokine is involved in internal anti-inflammatory and homeostatic processes. Thus, the bystander reaction mechanism both stimulates and controls inflammation.

Plant extracts of *Bellis perennis* (English Daisy), *Atropa belladonna* (Enchanter's Nightshade), and *Conium maculatum* (Poison Hemlock) were used by Heine and Schmolz in a dilution of one part in a hundred. They were mixed with whole blood cultures taken from healthy volunteers. The effects on macrophages and T cells in the blood were then examined. Plant materials had the same effect as other antigens on the immune response. "All three plant extracts tested proved capable of stimulating lymphocytes to release TGF-*beta*," wrote the authors. "Bellis perennis and Conium maculatum produced very distinct activity in all cases, while the effects of Atropa belladonna, although clearly weaker, must still be categorized as legitimately stimulatory" (Heine and Schmolz 1998).

Research on treatment through the use of the bystander reaction was summarized by Heine in 2007 (see his contributions in Pischinger 2007). Diluted antigens from nonplant sources have been administered orally, by aerosol, or by subcutaneous IV, with stimulative effects, so it can be supposed that plant extracts can be administered in the same ways.

Although the research of Heine and Schmolz confirms that small amounts of plant material act like antigens on the bystander immune system, they did not determine a strategy for using them in the treatment of illness, so Heine suggested a mechanism. Since T cells respond to precise protein "motifs," herbs used in small doses may possess related motifs in order to produce a relevant immunological response. In other words, the plant materials may possess motifs of their own resembling those in the T cells involved in the inflammatory reaction. This suggested to Heine the homeopathic "law of similars" as a basis for therapy (see his contributions to Pischinger 2007).

At the time he undertook this research, Heine was associated with the Heel Corporation in Germany, which makes Traumeel and other herbal and homeopathic preparations that use small doses of plant extracts. It is therefore clear that he had a vested interest in uncovering a scientific mechanism for the use of these preparations. At any rate, this is a start toward a pharmacological explanation that is not based on the structure/function claim, or artificial manipulation of the organism, but on the use of small amounts of a natural substance to cause a curative, immune-based, self-healing reaction in the body.

The law of similars, in homeopathy, is based on the idea that a substance causes what it cures. If the antigen presented by the plant substance produces an immune reaction similar to the symptoms produced by a disease, the thinking is that it will stimulate a self-healing reaction against the offending toxin, microbe, or causative agent. This type of reaction has been studied in pharmacology.

The Regulatory, Reverse, and Rebound Effects

Over the years, even conventional pharmacology has become aware of the fact that large and small doses of the same drug can cause unexpected or even opposite reactions in different people or at different times. This is a matter of real concern in conventional medicine. Three mechanisms for this kind of reaction have been identified. They have been named the regulatory, rebound,* and reverse effects. A comprehensive review of research on these three mechanisms was compiled by Madeleine Bastide (1998). An excellent review of

---

*The term *rebound effect* is used in both pharmacology and economics. There is no relationship between the two applications.

hormesis, or the reverse effect, was undertaken by M. Oberbaum and J. Cambar (1994).

৯ Regulatory Effect

When a substance that is normally present in a cell is given in low amounts, it can act as a stimulant to biological activity, but when given in large amounts, it can inhibit activity and injure or kill the organism. This reaction is based on "mechanistic cybernetic regulation using signal-molecules"; that is, the substance increases cellular activity through its normal signaling capacity in a feedback loop. With this, we are "strictly in the cybernetic information network with a signal effect" (Bastide 1998, 12, 4); in other words, we are still operating by structure/function.

৯ Reverse Effect

An example of the reverse effect in an herb would be the opposite reactions to Valerian (*Valeriana officinalis*) that are often observed by herbalists. The same dose can act as a stimulant or a sedative in two different people, or a single person may react in an opposite fashion to different concentration levels.

The reverse effect is caused by substances that are not normally found in the organism and therefore do not have biological signaling capabilities, unlike those used in the regulatory effect. The organism is sensitive to the substance but it can react in different ways. Dilution by as little as a factor of one part in ten or a hundred can then cause an opposite reaction. This change is therefore due to concentration.

Because of the reverse effect, many "chemicals, alkaloids, metals, etc., are listed in manuals of Pharmacology with indications of the opposite effects observed as a function of concentration" (Bastide 1998, 6). This is also called *hormesis*. It is not considered a "law" but a widely observable and often unpredictable phenomenon. Hormesis has been demonstrated with "various poisons and on all possible organisms whatever their level in evolution, from prokaryotic cells to plants, from eukaryotic cells to mammals" (Bastide 1998, 6).

Hormesis can be applied to protect the organism against a bad reaction to a substance. If a small dose is taken in advance of the large one, especially repeatedly, it has been observed that the toxic reaction of the large dose will be reduced or eliminated. The classic example of this was the practice of King Mithridates, who took small doses of poisons until he became immune to all the common poisons of his day. Unfortunately, he was killed by a sword. "The protection is strictly given by identity between the pretreatment and the poison and is strictly specific" (Bastide 1998, 6). This is called *mithridatization*. It is the principle behind vaccination.

Hormesis explains how organisms gain resistance to drugs. "We can propose that the resistance of bacteria to antibiotics, the resistance of parasites, the resistance of malignant cells to antimitotic substances (multi drug resistance) could originate in the hormetic model," demonstrating a "real learning process depending on the informative recognition of these poisons" by the organism (Bastide 1998, 9).

Hormesis can be used therapeutically to build up resistance to common stressors. Gardeners use the principle in the spring to build resistance to cold by bringing plants out of the hothouse for short periods of time, building up their tolerance for cold. Herbs could conceivably act in the same way, building up resistance to the kinds of stress. This, however, has not been tested (Bastide 12; Oberbaum and Cambar 1994).

༂ Rebound Effect

The rebound effect is not due to changes in concentration but by the effect of a toxic exposure followed by the natural, self-healing of the body. The toxin produces a set of symptoms, then the reaction of the organism produces a second set of symptoms. The rebound effect is, therefore, based on the innate self-healing ability of the organism.

The rebound effect is seen as the attempt of the organism to reestablish the original state of homeostasis that existed before the drug was administered. It does not occur due to concentration changes and is observable over time, rather than at once, as is the case of the regulatory and reverse effects.

Unfortunately, this is not how the rebound effect is conceived in conventional biomedicine. The symptoms of self-cure are defined as the "withdrawal symptoms" when a drug is removed. This phrase redefines the rebound effect from self-cure to addiction. We see here, once again, the problem of perspective. From a holistic perspective, the rebound effect is actually a general law of self-healing.

> Self-recovery is also called the rebound effect and is the consequence of the immunosuppressive effect [of the stressor]. It is a biological phenomenon which exists as a function of time after a strong pharmacological or toxic effect. (Bastide 1998, 5)

The organism itself is attempting to correct the problem, and it "presents the opposite manifestations as a dynamic reaction against poisoning."

Bastide is careful to point out that Selye's general adaptation reaction is not usually part of the picture. "It is not related to a general immunological mechanism," except in response to an immunosuppressive therapy. It is a specific reaction, or as Selye would say, local. "This self-recovery is the reaction of the living body to aggression, and self-recovery uses the appropriate and specific tools to reach a new equilibrium after the aggression" (Bastide 1998, 5).

The rebound effect is the basis of the homeopathic principle of cure introduced by Samuel Hahnemann, the founder of homeopathy. He detected both an initial toxic action of the poison and the following self-healing reaction (Hahnemann 1996, paragraphs 59, 63, 64). In homeopathy, the former is called the "primary reaction"; the latter a "secondary reaction." The credit for this observation is pointed out by Bastide and other European pharmacologists but hard to find in American pharmacology.

In order to develop symptomology on which to make a prescription—by inducing the secondary reaction—Hahnemann introduced the practice of drug proving. The poison or toxin is given in large or sustained doses until symptoms are produced. The initial symptoms would be primary. These are joined, after a time, by secondary symptoms generated in the effort of self-recovery. For use as a homeopathic drug, the substance is then diluted to reduce the primary effects and administered on the basis of the symptomology generated in the provings. Both primary and secondary symptoms are used as the basis for prescription.

Because the substance produced both sickness and its cure, Hahnemann considered the basic "law" of healing to be the "law of similars." Unfortunately, the law of similars can be shown to have gotten mixed up with the regulatory and reverse effects (Bastide 1998; Oberbaum and Cambar 1994). It can also be observed that this could have been called the law of contraries by Hahnemann, because the poison is a contrary that, in the end, causes healing.

It is necessary to reduce the dosage to reduce the toxic or primary effect if a poison is being used. This is the practice in homeopathy, which largely uses poisons. What about herbs? The vast majority are nontoxic in culinary or medicinal dosages.

It is often noted that herbs act by what is deemed contrary, or "hot to cold." The stimulant is used to warm up the extremities or increase circualation while the sedative reduces excitation or overstimulation. It appears, therefore, that the herb is being used to antidote the primary symptoms *or* reinforce the secondary response. For this reason, it can be said that herbs act by contrary or similarity. It is only when an herb or drug reaches the level of concentration where it can suppress the native self-healing response of the organism that we initiate the structure/function response. This is very difficult to do with herbs, many of which are widely used as foods.

The bystander response mechanism also explains the healing capacity of herbs and the low dilutions of homeopathic poisons. It seems to be a mechanical explanation of the rebound effect, or the primal self-healing mechanism of the body.

We have wandered far from our study of the matrix, but a consideration of the subject would be incomplete without considering mechanisms of cure other than the structure/function approach that damages the GRS and the ECM.

We can see from the above recitation of facts that herbs could act according to the regulatory, rebound, and reverse effects. It also has to be stated that these three mechanisms do not always produce "opposite" effects but often just different effects due to concentration or reaction.

In the final analysis, both contraries and similars have to be considered valid explanations for the self-healing reaction of the organism. But since both are true, and yet opposite, we must come to a definition that encompasses both. This was the thinking of naturopathic medical doctor Henry Lindlahr. He suggested that the law of healing should be called the "law of action and reaction." We arrive, therefore, at the law of karma, or the law of cause and effect operating at the biological level. This, clearly, is encompassing and correct. The organism reacts to forces that reinforce or challenge it by opposition.

References

Ahn, R. 2017. "Financial Ties of Principal Investigators and Randomized Control Trial Outcomes: Cross Sectional Study." *British Medical Journal* 356 (January 17).

Alfano, Massimo, Fillippo Canducci, Manuela Nebuloni, Massimo Clementi, Francesco Montorsi, and Andrea Salonia. 2016. "The Interplay of Extracellular Matrix and Microbiome in Urothelial Bladder Cancer." *Nature Reviews Urology* 13, no. 2 (first published online December 15, 2015): 77–90.

Angell, Marcia. 2004 *The Truth about Drug Companies: How They Deceive Us and What To Do about It.* New York: Random House.

———. 2009. "Drug Companies & Doctors: A Story of Corruption." *The New York Review of Books magazine.* (January 15, 2009).

Ashor, Ammar W., Jose Lara, John C. Mathers, and Mario Siervo. 2014. "Effect of Vitamin C on Endothelial Function in Health and Disease: A Systematic Review and Meta-analysis of Randomised Controlled Trials." *Atherosclerosis* 235, no. 1 (July): 9–20.

Barefoot, Robert R. and Carl Reich. 2002. *The Calcium Factor: The Scientific Secret of Health and Youth.* Wickenburg, Ariz.: Bokar Consultants.

Barnard, Julian. 1981. *Bach Flower Remedies: Form and Function.* Hudson, N.Y.: Steiner Books.

Barnes, Broda O., and Lawrence Galton. 1976. *Hypothyroidism: The Unsuspected Illness.* New York: Harper.

Bastide, M. 1998. "Basic Research on High Dilution Effects." In *High Dilution Effects on Cells and Integrated Systems,* edited by Paolo Marotta and Cloe

Taddei-Ferretti, 3–15. River Edge, N.J., and London: World Scientific Publishing Co. Pte. Ltd.

Bauman, Hannah, and Ashley Schmidt. 2015. "Food as Medicine; Prickly Pear Cactus (Opuntia ficus-indica, Cactaceae)." *Herbal Gram* 12, no. 9 (September).

Bergner, Paul. 1997. "Alteratives and Bad Blood." *Medical Herbalism* 8, no. 4 (January 31): 13.

Bernard, Claude. 1980. *An Introduction to the Study of Experimental Medicine.* Facsimile of the 1927 edition. Birmingham, Ala.: The Classics of Medicine Society.

Card, Dallas, and Shashank Srivastava. 2014. "Summary and Discussion of: 'Why Most Published Research Findings Are False.'" Statistics Journal Club 36-825 (December 10): 1–15.

Castillo, Diego J., Riaann F. Rifkin, Don A. Cowan, and Marnie Potgieter. 2019. "The Healthy Human Blood Microbiome: Fact or Fiction?" *Frontiers in Cellular and Infection Microbiology* 9 (May 8): 148.

Chu, Wing-kwan, Sabrina C. M. Cheung, Roxanna A. W. Lau, and Iris F. F. Benzie. 2011. "Bilberry (*Vaccinium myrtillus* L.)." In *Herbal Medicine: Biomolecular and Clinical Aspects,* 2nd ed., edited by I. F. F. Benzie and S. Wachtel-Galor, 55–72. Boca Raton, La.: CRC Press/Taylor & Francis.

Clarke, John Henry. 1886. *Indigestion: Its Causes and Cure.* Philadelphia: Boericke & Tafel.

Clymer, R. Swinburne. 1963. *Nature's Healing Agents.* Quakertown, Penn.: published by Clymer.

Cooper, Steven J. 2008. "From Claude Bernard to Walter Cannon: Emergence of the Concept of Homeostasis." *Appetite* 51, no. 3 (November): 419–27.

Cowan, Thomas S., and Sally Fallon Morrell. 2020. *The Contagion Myth; Why Viruses (including "Coronavirus") Are Not the Cause of Disease.* New York: Skyhorse Publishing.

Crellin, J. K., and J. Philpot. 1990. *Herbal Medicine Past and Present.* Vol. I, *Trying to Give Ease.* Durham, N.C., and London: Duke University Press.

Cutting, Keith. 2011. "Wound Healing through Synergy of Hyaluronan and an Iodine Complex." *Journal of Wound Care* 20, no. 9 (September): 424, 426, 428–30.

Davidson, William M. 1979. *A Series of Eight Special Lectures on Medical Astrology and Health.* Edited by Vivia Jayne. Monroe, N.Y.: Published by the Astrological Bureau.

Davis, Nicole. 2018. "The Human Microbiome: Why Our Microbes Could Be Key to Our Health." *Guardian,* March 26.

Dongari-Bagtzoglou, Anna. 2008. "Pathogenesis of Mucosal Biofilm Infections: Challenges and Progress." *Expert Review of Anti-infective Therapy* 6, no. 2 (April): 201–8.

d'Uscio, Livius V., Sheldon Milstein, Darcy Richardson, Leslie Smith, and Zvonimir S. Katusic. 2002. "Long-Term Vitamin C Treatment Increases Vascular Tetrahydrogiopterin Levels and Nitric Oxide Synthase Activity." *Circulation Research* 92, no. 1 (December 2): 88–95.

Elsen, Jonathan. 2015. "What Does the Term Microbiome Mean? Where Did It Come From? A Bit of a Surprise." *microBEnet* (April 8).

Felter, Harvey Wickes. 1910. *John Milton Scudder, M.D.* A Serial Publication of the Lloyd Library. Cincinnati, Ohio: Southwest School of Botanical Medicine.

———. 1922. "The Evolution of Specific Medication." *Eclectic Medical Journal* 82: 5873–80. Cincinnati, Ohio: Published by John K. Scudder, M.D.

Ferril, William B. *The Body Heals.* 2004. Whitefish, Mont.: Bridge Medical Publishers.

Firstenberg, Arthur. 2016. *The Invisible Rainbow: The History of Electricity and Life.* Washington, D.C.: AGB Press.

Fouad, Yousef Ahmed and Carmen Aanei. "Revisiting the Hallmarks of Cancer." *Am J Cancer Res.* 7, no. 5 (May 1, 2017): 1016–36.

Frantz, Christian, Kathleen M. Stewart, and Valerie M. Weaver. 2010. "The Extracellular Matrix at a Glance." *Journal of Cell Science* 123, part 24 (December 15): 4195–4200.

Freedman, David H. "Lies, Damned Lies, and Medical Science." *Atlantic,* November 2010.

Friedman, A., and H. L. Weiner. 1994. "Induction of Anergy or Active Suppression Following Oral Tolerance Is Determined by Antigen." *Proceedings of the National Academy of Sciences of the United States of America* 91, no. 14 (July 5): 6688–92.

Fujimura, K. E., T. Demoor, M. Rauch, A. A. Farugi, S. Jang, C. C. Johnson, H. A. Boushey, et al. 2014. "House Dust Exposure Mediates Gut Microbiome *Lactobacillus* Enrichment and Airway Immune Defense against Allergens and Virus Infection," *Proceedings of the National Academy of Sciences of the United States of America* 111, no. 2 (January 14): 805–10.

Fulton, John F., and Leonard G. Wilson, compilers. 1966. *Selected Readings in the History of Physiology.* 2nd ed. Springfield, Ill.: Charles C Thomas.

Gillies R. J., C. Pilot, Y. Marunaka, and S. Fais. 2019. "Targeting Acidity in Cancer and Diabetes." *Biochim Biophys Acta Rev Cancer.* 1871 no. 2 (April): 273–80.

Gohil, Kashmira J., Jagruti A. Patel, and Anuradha K. Gajjar. 2010. "Pharmacological Review on *Centella asiatica:* A Potential Herbal Cure-all." *Indian Journal of Pharmaceutical Sciences* 72, no. 5 (September–October): 546–56.

Gøtzsche, P. C. 2012. "Big Pharma Often Commits Corporate Crime, and This Must Be Stopped." *British Medical Journal* 345 (December 14).

Gross, Charles. 1998. "Claude Bernard and the Constancy of the Internal Environment." *Neuroscientist.* 4, no. 5 (September 1): 380–85.

Groves, Philip W. 2004. *Science and Esoteric Wisdom.* Sydney: Triune Publishing.

Gümbel, Dietrich. 1993. *Principles of Holistic Therapy with Herbal Essences.* Brussels: Haug International.

Guyton, Arthur C. 1976. *Textbook of Medical Physiology.* 5th ed. Philadelphia: W. B. Saunders.

Hahnemann, Samuel. 1996. *Organon of the Medical Art.* Edited by Wendy Reilly. Redmond, Wash.: Birdcage Books.

Hakomori, Senitiroh. 2002. "Glycosylation Defining Cancer Malignancy: New Wine in an Old Bottle." *PNAS* 99 no. 16 (August 6): 10231–33.

Hall, Dorothy. 1991. *Dorothy Hall's Herbal Medicine.* Sydney, Melbourne, and Auckland: Lothian Publishing Company Pty. Ltd.

Haller, John. 1999. *A Profile in Alternative Medicine: The Eclectic Medical College of Cincinnati, 1845–1942.* Kent, Ohio: Kent State University Press.

Healthline website. "Immunodeficiency Disorders."

Heine, Hartmut, and Manfred Schmolz. 1998. "Induction of the Immunological Bystander Reaction by Plant Extracts." *Biomedical Therapy* XVI, no. 3 (February): 12–14.

Horne, Steven. 2009. "Applied Lymphology: Unlocking the Secret to Pain Relief." The School of Modern Herbal Medicine website.

Horton, Richard. 2015. "Offline: What Is Medicine's 5 Sigma?" *Lancet* 385, no. 9976 (April 11): 1380.

Howell, Edward. 1985. *Enzyme Nutrition.* New York: Avery Publishing.

Hyiodine website. 2019, 2021. "Woundhealing with Hyaluronic Acid Works Well on Humans and Pets."

Hynes, Richard O., and Alexandra Naba. 2011. "Overview of the Matrisome—An Inventory of Extracellular Matrix Constituents and Functions." *Cold Spring Harbor Perspectives in Biology 4,* no. 1 (September).

Ioannidis, John. 2005. "Why Most Published Research Findings Are False." *PLOS Medicine* 2, no. 8 (August 30): e124.

———. 2016. "The Mass Production of Redundant, Misleading, and Conflicted Systematic Reviews and Meta-analysis." *Milbank Quarterly* 94, no. 3 (September): 485–514.

Israel, Barbara A., and Warren I. Schaeffer. 1988. "Cytoplasmic Mediation of Malignancy." *In Vitro Cellular & Developmental Biology* 24, no. 5 (May): 487–90.

Jerosch, Jörg. 2011. "Effects of Glucosamine and Chondroitin Sulfate on Cartilage Metabolism in OA: Outlook on Other Nutrient Partners Especially Omega-3 Fatty Acids." *International Journal of Rheumatology* 2011: 969012.

Juschten, Jenny, Pieter Tuinman, Nicole Juffermans, Barry Dixon, Marcel Levi, and Marcus Schultz. "Nebulized Anticoagulants in Lung Injury in Critically Ill Patients: An Updated Systematic Review of Preclinical and Clinical Studies." *Annals of Translational Medicine* 5, no. 22 (November 2017): 444.

Kaltreider, Nolan L., George R. Meneely, James R. Allen, and William F. Bale. 1941. "Determination of the Volume of the Extracellular Fluid of the Body with Radioactive Sodium." *Journal of Experimental Medicine* 74, no. 6 (November 30): 569–90.

Kendrick, Malcolm. 2013. "If Not Cholesterol, What?" Dr. Malcolm Kendrick website, November 3.

Keown, Daniel. 2014. *The Spark in the Machine: How the Science of Acupuncture Explains the Mysteries of Western Medicine.* London: Singing Dragon.

Korr, Irvin M. 1997. *The Collected Papers of Irvin M. Korr.* Vol. 2. Indianapolis, Ind.: American Academy of Osteopathy.

Kresser, Chris. 2016. "Biofilm: What It Is and How to Treat It." Kresser Institute website, March 6.

Liubakka, Alyssa, and Byron P. Vaughn. 2016. "Clostridium Difficile Infection and Fecal Microbiota Transplant," *AACN Advanced Critical Care* 27, no. 3 (July): 324–37.

Lopez, D. A., R. M. Williams, and K. Miehlke. 1994. *Enzymes: The Fountain of Life.* 1st English ed. Mt. Pleasant, S.C.: Neville Press.

Luciani, Luigi. 1911. *Human Physiology: Circulation and Respiration.* Vol. 1. London: Macmillan and Co., Limited.

Marinelli, Ralph, Branko Fuerst, Hoyte van der Zee, Andrew McGinn, William Marinelli, James D. Stewart, and Michael Duffy. 1995. "The Heart Is Not a Pump: A Refutation of the Pressure Propulsion Premise of Heart Function." *Frontier Perspectives* 5, no. 1 (Fall–Winter).

Marunaka, Yoshinori. 2015. "Roles of Interstitial Fluid pH in Diabetes Mellitus: Glycolysis and Mitochondrial Function." *World Journal of Diabetes* 6, no. 1 (February 15): 125–35.

Maury, Marguerite. 1996. *Marguerite Maury's Guide to Aromatherapy.* London: Random House.

Moore, Michael. 1989. *Medicinal Plants of the Desert and Canyon West.* Santa Fe: Museum of New Mexico.

Myers, Tom. 2018. "Interstitium: A Statement from Tom Myers." Anatomy Trains website, March 29.

Naviaux, Robert K. 2014. "Metabolic Features of the Cell Danger Response." *Mitochondrion* 16 (May): 7–17.

———. 2019. "Metabolic Features and Regulation of the Healing Cycle—A New Model for Chronic Disease Pathogenesis and Treatment." *Mitochondrion* 46 (May): 278–97.

Newman, Tim. 2017. "High Blood Pressure: Sodium May Not Be the Culprit." *Medical News Today* website, April 26.

Oberbaum, M. and J. Cambar. 1994. "Hormesis: Dose-Dependent Reverse Effects of Low and Very Low Doses." In *Ultra High Dilution: Physiology and Physics,* edited by P. C. Endler and J. Schulte, 5–18. Vienna: Springer, Science+Business Media, BV.

Olczyk, Pawel, Łukasz Mencner, Katarzyna Komosinksa-Vassev. 2014. "The Role of the Extracellular Matrix Components in Cutaneous Wound Healing." *BioMed Research International.*

Oshman, James L. 2016. *Energy Medicine: The Scientific Basis.* London: Churchill Livingston Elsevier.

Overton, Elliot. 2018. "Sulfate II: The Living Matrix and Structured Water." Elliot Overton Nutrition & Functional Medicine website, September 19.

Pasupuleti, Visweswara Rao, Lakhsmi Sammugam, Nagesvari Ramesh, and Siew Hua Gan. 2017. "Honey, Propolis, and Royal Jelly: Comprehensive Review of Their Biological Actions and Health Benefits." *Oxidative Medicine and Cellular Longevity* 2017 (July 26).

Pischinger, Alfred. 1991. *Matrix and Matrix Regulation: Basis for a Holistic Theory of Medicine.* English translation by N. MacLean. Edited by Hartmut Heine. Brussels: Editions Haug International. Originally published in 1975.

———. 2007. *The Extracellular Matrix and Ground Regulation: Basis for a Holistic Biological Medicine.* Edited by Harmut Heine. Berkeley, Calif.: North Atlantic Books.

Pollack, Gerald H. 2001. *Cells, Gels, and the Engines of Life.* Seattle, Wash.: Ebner and Sons.

———. 2015. "The Fourth Phase of Water." *Wise Traditions in Food, Farming, and the Healing Arts,* Winter issue. Available at the Weston A. Price Foundation website.

Prashanth, L., K. K. Kattapagari, R. T. Chitturi, V. R. R. Baddam, and L. K. Prasad. 2015. "A Review on Role of Essential Trace Elements in Health and Disease." *Journal of Dr. NTR University of Health Sciences* 4, no. 2: 75–85.

Princeton University. 2019 "Plants and Microbes Shape Global Biomes through Local Underground Alliances." Press release. *Science Daily,* April 17.

Ramsey, James M. 1982. *Basic Pathophysiology: Modern Stress and the Disease Process.* Boston: Addison-Wesley Educational Publishers Inc.

Rattle, Simon, Oliver Hofmann, Christopher P. Price, Larry J. Kricka, and David Wild. 2013. "Lab-on-a-Chip, Micro- and Nanoscale Immunoassay Systems, and Microarrays." In *The Immunoassay Handbook,* 4th ed., edited by David Wild. Amsterdam: Elsevier.

Rettner, Rachael. 2018. "Meet Your Interstitium, a Newfound "Organ." Scientific American website, March 27.

Salih, B., T. Sipahi, and E. Oybak Dönmez. 2009. "Ancient Nigella Seeds from Boyalı Höyük in North-Central Turkey." *Journal of Ethnopharmacology* 124, no. 3 (July 30): 416–20.

Schierwagen, Robert, Camila Alvarez-Silva, Mette Simone Aae Madsen, Carl Christian Kolbe, Carsten Meyer, Daniel Thomas, Frank Erhard Uschner, et al. 2019. "Circulating Microbiome in Blood of Different Circulatory Compartments." *Gut* 68, no. 3: 578–80.

Schmidt, Richard J. 2003. Review of *Cells, Gels, and the Engines of Life,* by Gerald H. Pollack. *Journal of Pharmacy and Pharmacology* 55: 857–58.

Schoenfeld, Jonathan D., and John P. A. Ioannidis. 2013. "Is Everything We Eat Associated with Cancer? A Systematic Cookbook Review." *American Journal of Clinical Nutrition* 97, no. 1: 127–34.

Schüessler, Wilhelm Heinrich. 1898. *An Abridged Therapy: Manual for the Biochemical Treatment of Disease.* Philadelphia: Boericke & Tafel.

Scudder, John M. 1870. *Specific Medication and Specific Medicine.* Cincinnati, Ohio: Wilstach, Baldwin, & Co., Printers.

———. 1874. *Specific Diagnosis.* Cincinnati, Ohio: Wilstach, Baldwin, & Co.

———. 1898. *American Eclectic Materia Medica and Therapeutics.* 12th ed. Cincinnati, Ohio: The Scudder Brothers Company, Publishers.

———. 1997. "The John M. Scudder Organ Remedies, 1892–3." Edited by Francis Brinker. Special issue, *Eclectic Medical Journal* 2, no. 6.

Selye, Hans. 1956. *The Stress of Life.* New York, Toronto, London: MacGraw-Hill Book Company.

Shook, Edward. 1978. *Advanced Treatise on Herbology.* Trinity Center Press.

Sofat, Nidhi, Robin Wait, Saralili D. Robertson, Deborah L. Baines, and Emma H. Baker. 2015. "Interaction between Extracellular Matrix Molecules and Microbial Pathogens: Evidence for the Missing Link in Autoimmunity with Rheumatoid Arthritis as a Disease Model," *Frontiers in Microbiology* 5, no. 783 (January 14).

Spittle, Constance R. 1974. "The Effect of Vitamin C on the Blood Vessels." *Proceedings of the Journal of Clinical Pathology* 27, no. 6 (June): 513.

St. John, Ashley L., and Soman N. Abraham. 2013. "Innate Immunity and Its Regulation by Mast Cells." *Journal of Immunology* 190, no. 9 (May 1): 4458–63.

Surjushe, Amar, Resham Vasani, and D. G. Saple. 2008. "Aloe Vera: A Short Review." *Indian Journal of Dermatology* 53, no. 4: 163–66.

Tassell, Mary. 2013. *Posology in Herbal Medicine: Do We Have a Sound Basis?* M.S. dissertation, Scottish School of Herbal Medicine, accredited by the University of Wales.

Teplicki, Eric, Qianli Ma, David E. Castillo, Mina Zarei, Adam P. Hustad, Juan Chen, and Jie Li. 2018. "The Effects of Aloe Vera on Wound Healing in Cell Proliferation, Migration, and Viability." *Wounds* 30, no. 9: 263–68.

Thurston, Joseph. 1900. *The Philosophy of Physiomedicalism.* Richmond, Ind.: Published by Thurston.

Tran, Q., H. Lee, C. Kim, G. Kong, N. Gong, S. H. Kwon, J. Park, S. H. Kim, and J. Park. 2020. "Revisiting the Warburg Effect: Diet-Based Strategies for Cancer Prevention." *Biomed Res Int.* (August 4).

Virchow, Rudolf. 1971. *Cellular Pathology.* English translation. New York: Dover Publications.

Weiner, H. L., and F. Meyer. 1996. "Oral Tolerance: Mechanisms and Applications." *Annals of the New York Academy of Sciences* 778: 1–418.

West, C. Samuel. 1981. *The Golden Seven Plus One.* 1st ed. Orem, Utah: Samuel Publishing.

White, George S. 1939. *The Finer Forces of Nature in Diagnosis and Therapy.* Los Angeles, Calif.: Self-published.

Williams, Roger J. 1977. Biochemical Individuality. Austin: University of Texas Press.

Windsor, W. Jon. 2020. "How Quorum Sensing Works." American Society for Microbiology website, June 12.

Wood, Matthew. 2000. *Vitalism: History of Herbalism, Homeopathy, and the Flower Essences.* Berkeley, Calif.: North Atlantic Books.

Wood, Matthew, Francis Bonaldo, and Phyllis Light. 2016. *Traditional Western Herbalism and Pulse Evaluation: A Conversation.* Morrisville, N.C.: Lulu Publishing.

Worcester, John. 1889. *Physiological Correspondences.* Reprint. West Chester, Penn.: the Swedenborg Foundation, 2009.

Yang, Joy. 2012. "The Human Microbiome Project: Extending the Definition of What Constitutes a Human." National Human Genome Research Institute website, July 16.

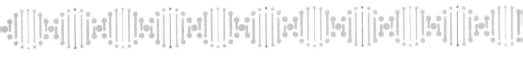

Index

BOOKS OF RELATED INTEREST

Adaptogens
Herbs for Strength, Stamina, and Stress Relief
by David Winston, RH(AHG)
with Steven Maimes

Medical Herbalism
The Science and Practice of Herbal Medicine
by David Hoffmann, FNIMH, AHG

The Herbal Handbook
A User's Guide to Medical Herbalism
by David Hoffmann, FNIMH, AHG

Natural Antibiotics and Antivirals
18 Infection-Fighting Herbs and Essential Oils
by Christopher Vasey, N.D.

Plant Intelligence and the Imaginal Realm
Beyond the Doors of Perception into the Dreaming of Earth
by Stephen Harrod Buhner

Liberating Yourself from Lyme
An Integrative and Intuitive Guide to Healing Lyme Disease
by Vir McCoy and Kara Zahl

Energetic Cellular Healing and Cancer
Treating the Emotional Imbalances at the Root of Disease
by Tjitze de Jong
Foreword by Robert Holden, Ph.D.

The Body Clock in Traditional Chinese Medicine
Understanding Our Energy Cycles for Health and Healing
by Lothar Ursinus

INNER TRADITIONS • BEAR & COMPANY
P.O. Box 388
Rochester, VT 05767
1-800-246-8648
www.InnerTraditions.com

Or contact your local bookseller